Francisco Diéguez Quesada

Educational program to prevent chronic kidney disease

Francisco Diéguez Quesada

Educational program to prevent chronic kidney disease

in patients with type 2 diabetes mellitus

ScienciaScripts

Imprint

Cover image: www.ingimage.com

This book is a translation from the original published under ISBN 978-613-9-44135-8.

Publisher:
Sciencia Scripts
is a trademark of
Dodo Books Indian Ocean Ltd. and OmniScriptum S.R.L publishing group

120 High Road, East Finchley, London, N2 9ED, United Kingdom
Str. Armeneasca 28/1, office 1, Chisinau MD-2012, Republic of Moldova, Europe
Printed at: see last page
ISBN: 978-620-8-31886-4

Contents

AUTHORS: Dr. Francisco Dieguez Quesada
DrC. Rafael Enrique Cruz Abascal.
Dr. Alleiny Aurora Perez Ram^ez
Dr. Diana Rosa Gonzalez Garrta
Dr. Felix Felipe Sosa Guardado
Lic in Nursing Santiago Luis Gamoneda Perez

"If someone desires good health, he must first ask himself whether he is ready to eliminate the reasons for his illness. Only then is it possible to help him.

Hippocrates

DEDICATION

To my parents, who throughout my life taught me to strive for my goals and encouraged me to keep moving forward.
To my wife, because without her support, understanding and dedication I would not have reached the goal I have reached today.
To my children for being my inspiration to achieve everything.
To all those who have supported me in becoming what I am.

ACKNOWLEDGEMENTS

To all those who in one way or another offered me their support, help and guidance, without which the completion of this work would not have been possible.

- Ami tutor.
- Ami adviser.
- To my teachers in the teachers.
- Amis friends for their support unconditional support.
- To the health staff and patients of CMF 47 and 48 who collaborated and without whom I would not have been able to carry out this study.

SUMMARY

Chronic Kidney Disease (CKD) is a common complication of Diabetes Mellitus. Early diagnosis decreases disease progression, improves quality of life and increases life expectancy. **Objective: To** determine the efficacy of an educational programme to prevent CKD in patients with type 2 diabetes mellitus. **Method**: A pre-experimental, prospective, intervention study was carried out in two family doctor's offices of the XX Aniversario polyclinic, Santa Clara municipality, in the period between June 2022 and March 2024. With a population of 177 diabetic patients, the sample consisted of 60 of them, selected with a non-probabilistic intentional sampling, which fulfilled the inclusion criteria. **Results**: 53.3% of the sample studied were in the age range of 60 to 79 years, 68.3% were female, 43.3% had pre-university education and 40% were overweight. Dyslipidaemia (85%), hypertension (73.3%) and smoking (31.7%) were the main risk factors for developing CKD. There was a predominance of positive albuminuria (58.3%) and it was more frequent in patients with more than 6 years of DM. The level of information before the educational action was low, rising after its application in more than 90% of the sample. **Conclusions**: The educational programme was effective in raising the information level of type 2 diabetic patients to prevent CKD.

Keywords: Diabetes Mellitus, Chronic Kidney Disease, risk factors.

CHAPTER 1

INTRODUCTION

Diabetes mellitus (DM) is one of the most common chronic non-communicable diseases and therefore one of the fastest growing health emergencies in recent decades, and is now considered one of the major health problems worldwide.[1] According to the World Health Organization (WHO), the number of people with diabetes worldwide is reported to have increased from 30 million in 1995 to 347 million people today and is estimated to reach 366 million by 2030. According to the International Diabetes Federation (IDF), China, India, the United States, Brazil, Russia and Mexico are, in that order, the countries with the highest number of diabetics. However, the incidence and prevalence of the disease is growing every day in both developed and developing countries, although there are significant differences.[3,4]

Recent studies have shown that there is a predominant incidence of type 2 DM; it is described as affecting not only adults, but can also occur early in life. The worldwide prevalence of this clinical form has increased from 4.7% to 8.5% in the adult population in the last two decades. [5]

One of the most frequent chronic complications in diabetic patients is diabetic kidney disease (DKD). It is estimated at 150 to 200 million and it is estimated that 30% to 50% of adults with type 2 DM have renal involvement from the time of diagnosis, which is a marker of prognosis and quality of life and one third of them may progress to advanced stages of chronic kidney disease (CKD). [6, 7,8]

CKD is one of the most common and devastating complications of type 2 DM, with no expectation of cure or remission, it is of rapid and progressive evolution, it triggers various reactions for patients and affects their quality of life. The epidemiological view of this disease has undergone a remarkable change in the last twenty years, nowadays it affects a significant percentage of the population and is related to phenomena or diseases of high prevalence, such as DM[9--101112]

This disease is a major problem worldwide, which is why it is important to prevent its occurrence and avoid the development of complications. In the United States, Canada and Japan, between 8 and 11% of the adult population suffers from this condition. ' ' [1314] In Mexico, there is an estimated incidence of 377 cases per million inhabitants, with an estimated 52,000 patients in substitutive therapies. Similarly, Argentina has had for many years a sustained growth in the prevalence of patients on renal replacement therapy. [15,16]

There are several strategies in the world to detect it in a simple way at the first level of care. In high-risk groups (DM, hypertension, dyslipidaemia or systemic vascular damage) they are all based on an intentional search for risk factors, including the determination of markers of renal damage.[11] These are albuminuria, proteinuria, Addis count, creatinine and glomerular filtration rate, among others. [17, 18,19]

Between 25-40% of diabetic patients will have some degree of nephropathy during the course of their disease, the prevalence of which will depend on numerous factors involved in its pathogenesis (genetics, time course of diabetes, degree of glycaemic control, adequate or inadequate blood pressure management, dyslipidaemia, smoking, onset of albuminuria and progression to proteinuria), which will mark the progression to DRE. [20,21]

Its prevalence is steadily increasing mainly in less developed countries. The risk of mortality in DRD increases by 31.1% and imposes an enormous human, economic and social burden. The diagnosis of RDE is often made at an advanced stage because of limited knowledge and the absence of early diagnosis programmes. ' '. [2223] Hence the importance of early detection and treatment, as it is the leading cause of advanced kidney disease.

In our country there is a National Diabetic Care Programme, whose fundamental activities are carried out at all levels of care, although a large part of them correspond to the primary level of care due to its great weight in health promotion and prevention actions, which advocates healthy lifestyles, as well as actions for the detection of the disease and its potential acute and chronic complications. To this end, the training of health care providers, patients and their families at all levels of the system is of paramount importance. Diabetes Care Centres (DACs) have an important role to play in this context. Diabetes education and control of glycaemia and vascular risk factors are essential elements of the programme's strategy.

Cuba has a prevalence of DM higher than the rate of 60 per 1000 inhabitants. In Villa Clara, 6.5 % of the total population suffers from this disease and most cases are diagnosed when the disease has progressed. According to the author, since CKD is one of the most common and devastating complications of type 2 DM, it is necessary for prevention in Primary Health Care (PHC) to adopt an active approach, so that the population is informed of the magnitude of the problem of DM and CKD, and the need for changes in healthy lifestyles should be promoted and disseminated among the high-risk population. [24]

The XX Aniversario polyclinic, where this research was carried out, has 8.3 % of its population diagnosed with type 2 DM and in the family medical offices 47 and 48, 8.4% have this disease and of these, 30.7% have CKD.

CHAPTER 2

SCIENTIFIC PROBLEM

Because DM and CKD are diseases that represent a major public health problem, they are resource-intensive and require an adequate coordination of the various public and private sectors in order to be tackled.

professionals involved in their care, the following question arises scientific:

How to decrease the occurrence of CKD in patients with type 2 DM who belong to the family medical offices 47 and 48 of the XX Aniversario polyclinic, in the period between June 2022 and March 2024?

HYPOTHESIS

The implementation of an educational programme will strengthen the information level of patients with type 2 DM about CKD and contribute to decrease the risk factors for CKD.

OBJECTIVES

GENERAL OBJECTIVE

To determine the effectiveness of an educational programme to prevent CKD in patients with type 2 DM.

SPECIFIC OBJECTIVES

1. To characterise patients with type 2 DM according to sociodemographic and clinical variables of interest.
2. To identify albuminuria as an early marker of renal damage in patients with type 2 DM participating in the study.
3. Design the educational programme to prevent CKD in patients with type 2 DM.
4. To assess the level of information about CKD in the study sample before and after the educational intervention.

CHAPTER 3

THEORETICAL FRAMEWORK

DM is a metabolic disorder of multiple aetiology characterised by chronic hyperglycaemia, accompanied by disorders of carbohydrate, fat and protein metabolism, caused by defects in insulin secretion, insulin peripheral action or both. It presents with characteristic symptoms such as thirst, polyuria, weight loss or blurred vision, which may progress to ketoacidosis, hyperosmolarity, stupor, coma and death if not effectively treated. However, hyperglycaemia can evolve for years leading to late complications before the diagnosis of DM is made.

Complications of DM can be specific, diabetic microangiopathy such as retinopathy which can lead to vision loss, nephropathy which can progress to advanced renal failure and/or neuropathy with risk of ulcers and amputations, Charcot's joint, neurovegetative dysfunction, including sexual dysfunction. In addition, people with diabetes are at increased risk of atherosclerosis, with manifestations of cardiovascular complications, such as, cardiac infarction, peripheral vascular insufficiency (amputations) and cerebrovascular disease (cerebrovascular accidents). 25

DM is today a growing health problem for both the developed and developing world. In 2000 there were already 165 million people with diabetes and 300 million are expected by 2025. People with diabetes have a reduced life expectancy and twice the mortality rate of the general population.

Improved DM care would increase the life expectancy of these people, but this in turn would lead to a higher incidence of micro-vascular (nephropathy and retinopathy) and macro-vascular (coronary heart disease, cerebrovascular and peripheral vascular disease) complications as age and duration of DM are the main uncontrollable risk factors, It will therefore be necessary to apply existing knowledge or develop technologies capable of preventing the onset of the disease and its complications, thus helping to reduce the economic burden on society, which is mainly concentrated on hospitalisation costs due to complications. 2[,627]

Classification of MD

There are different types of DM, as well as related disorders, which differ in their cause, clinical course and treatment. The main classifications are:

> Type 1 DM: usually appears in childhood or adolescence, although it can appear at any age. In most cases, endogenous insulin production disappears almost completely due to immune destruction of insulin-secreting cells and exogenous insulin is required to control glycaemia, prevent ketoacidosis and sustain life.

> Type 2 DM is a chronic disease that nowadays occurs more frequently in adults aged 50-55 years and is therefore called adult-onset diabetes. However, the diagnosis of this pathology in children and adolescents is becoming more and more frequent, due to the recent alarming increase in childhood obesity, a product of the sedentary lifestyle that has been adopted in recent years, especially observed in the western countries of the USA and Spain, where 18.2% of children and adolescents are diagnosed with type 2 diabetes.Its main characteristic is the presence of high blood glucose levels which is one of the main risk factors for cardiovascular diseases, so much so that if not treated properly, very serious complications such as

myocardial infarction can occur,
neurological diseases, diseases that can lead to blindness, amputation of the foot, etc. It is a chronic, lifelong disease characterised by high blood sugar (glucose) levels and is the most common form of diabetes.

> Gestational diabetes: usually occurs in either the second or third trimester of pregnancy in women who have never had a previous diagnosis of DM. The rise in glycaemia occurs between 24 and 28 weeks of pregnancy and is a high risk factor for complications during this period. This is due to the fact that during gestation there are important changes in the whole metabolism, because the foetal product requires a lot of energy from the mother in order to live and develop, such as nutrition, oxygen, the immune system, among others. The wear and tear that the mother suffers to maintain the development of the foetus, shows a simultaneous wear and tear and a deficit of insulin, and it is in this situation that the disease can appear. [28,29]

Risk factors associated with developing type 2 diabetes mellitus

Type 2 DM is a multifactorial disease involving both genetic and environmental factors as well as family history. However, factors such as low activity levels, poor diet and excess weight (especially around the waist) significantly increase the risk of developing type 2 DM. Other known risk factors include ethnicity (African Americans, Hispanic Americans and Native Americans have high rates of DM), age over 45, glucose intolerance, hypertension and a history of gestational diabetes. The main cause of type 2 DM is lifestyle related. It is poor diet leading to obesity, inactivity and sedentary lifestyles. 27, 30, 31, [32]

The risk factors for type 2 DM are divided into two groups:

I. Modifiable.

> Overweight and obesity
> Sedentary lifestyle
> Metabolic syndrome
> Arterial hypertension
> Dyslipidaemia
> Dietary factors

II. Not modifiable.

> Race
> Family history
> Age
> Sex
> History of gestational diabetes

Risk factors for the development of type 2 DM can be modified when identified early. Inadequate dietary habits, overweight, sedentary lifestyle, dyslipidaemia, AHT and genetic factors are the basis for insulin resistance and the metabolic syndrome that epidemiologically is affecting the world population, especially in Latin America. 33, 34, 35,

Diagnosis

The WHO and the International Diabetes Federation (IDF) recommend the following criteria.

> For diabetes: Fasting blood glucose greater than or equal to 7.0 mmol/l (126 mg/dl) or 11.1 mmol/l (200 mg/dl) at 2 h with an oral glucose load. Despite their

limitations, these criteria distinguish a group of patients with significantly increased premature mortality and risk of microvascular and cardiovascular complications.

> For pre-diabetes: Altered basal glucose (IFG) between 6.1-6.9 mmol/l fasting and blood glucose at 2 h after an oral load less than 7.8 mmol/l (140 mg/dl). The ADA lowered the fasting plasma glucose threshold to 5.6 mmol/l.

> Glucose tolerance disorder (GTD) if fasting blood glucose is less than 7.0 mmol/l (126 mg/dl) and at 2 h of an oral load greater than or equal to 7.8 and less than 11.1 mmol/l (140-200 mg/dl). 3'',[637 3839]

IFG and IGT are referred to as pre-diabetes, which is considered an intermediate state between normal blood glucose concentrations and those considered to be diabetic. Both categories are risk factors for diabetes and cardiovascular disease by unclear mechanisms, although it is known that the increased atherogenicity of these states is due to blood glucose disturbances. [38] The ADA recommends an oral glucose tolerance test with 100 g after a fast of at least 8 hours.

The diagnosis of gestational diabetes requires the determination of at least two of the following plasma glucose values in women: fasting > 5.3 mmol/l, one hour > 10.0 mmol/l, two hours > 8.6 mmol/l and three hours > 7.8 mmol/l. [3]8,3[9]

The ADA recommends screening for gestational DM when pregnancy is detected if any of these conditions are present: severe obesity, previous history of GDM or macrofetus delivery, glycosuria, polycystic ovary syndrome or family history of DM2. However, the WHO recommends universal screening for gestational DM for all women at 24-28 weeks gestation 1.

The WHO and IDF propose the oral glucose tolerance test as diagnostic because fasting plasma glucose misses about 30% of patients, identifies persons with IGT and often confirms or excludes impaired glucose tolerance in asymptomatic persons. This test should be used in persons with fasting blood glucose levels between 6.1 and 6.9 mmol/l (110-125 mg/dl) to determine glucose tolerance status. [39]

Diagnostic Methods

> Basal glycaemia in venous plasma (GBP): This method is the most recommended when seeking to diagnose type 2 DM and the execution of population studies. This is due to the fact that it is a highly accurate, low-cost, reproducible test that is easy to apply. In addition, it is known that measuring plasma glucose levels is about 11% higher than measured whole blood glucose, whether the test is given in a fasting or basal state. However, in non-basal (postprandial) states, the two are virtually identical.

> Oral glucose tolerance test (OGTT): This method is based on the identification of glycaemia levels in venous plasma, two hours after the patient (adult) has ingested 75 g of glucose. However, it is an approved test for the diagnosis of type 2 DM. Recommendations for its use are contradictory, as the American Diabetes Association (ADA) does not recommend it in routine practice, contrary to the WHO, which justifies its use to diagnose asymptomatic diabetes. In addition, this test is very poorly reproducible (due to difficult compliance in preparation), much more costly and uncomfortable for patients.

> Glycosylated haemoglobin (HbA1c): This method presents the average of blood glucose values over the last 3 months in a single evaluation and can be carried out at any time of the day, without the patient having to undergo prior preparation or fasting.

This test is highly recommended when seeking to control DM2. On the other hand, it has been thought that HbA1c would be useful in the diagnosis of diabetes in people with altered basal glycaemia (110-125 mg/dl), because, if a positive result is found in representation of a high specificity, or contradictory with a high sensitivity, it could avoid carrying out the creation of the curve. This would allow for an appropriate individualisation of treatments in this group of patients. ,[4041]

Criteria for good DM management

Glycosylated haemoglobin (HbA1c) is the best parameter of glycaemic control because it correlates with the occurrence of micro- and macrovascular complications in the long term and because it provides information on the degree of control in the previous 2-4 months. Epidemiological studies have shown that micro- and macrovascular complications increase at values above 8%. The European Consensus considers HbA1c of less than 6.5% as good control and HbA1c of less than 7.5% as acceptable; the ADA considers HbA1c of less than 7.5% as a therapeutic objective. In our country, a HbA1c of less than 7% is a target and therapeutic measures are intensified when HbA1c is higher than 8%. [42]

Achieving the haemoglobin A1c (HbA1c) target has been shown to be associated with reduced microvascular complications of diabetes mellitus when achieved early in the course of the disease. Studies have shown that chronic hyperglycaemia can cause a negative metabolic memory and increase the risk of chronic complications of diabetes; in contrast, subjects who achieve early glycaemic control have a positive "glycaemic legacy" that can extend its benefits over several years. Therefore, it is strongly recommended that the diabetes management plan be oriented towards early achievement of the therapeutic goal. While clinical practice guidelines recommend frequent monitoring of HbA1c.

Inadequate glycaemic control plays an important role in cardiovascular risk and diabetes remains the leading cause of blindness, kidney failure and non-traumatic lower limb amputations in the United States. The cornerstone of management of type 2 diabetes mellitus is to promote a lifestyle that includes a healthy diet, regular physical activity, smoking cessation and maintaining a healthy body weight. [4] [2,4] [3]

Complications

The key complications of MD are:

I. Acute

> Diabetic coma.
> Hyperosmolar coma.
> Lactic acidosis.
> Hypoglycaemic coma.
> Increased rate of acute infections

II. Chronicles

> MacroangiopaUa: Ischemic heart disease, stroke, heart failure encephalic vascular and peripheral vascular.
> MicroangiopaUa: diabetic retinopaUa, neuropaUas and ERD.

Diabetic Kidney Disease (DKD)

DRE is a problem of glomerular fibrosis and sclerosis secondary to haemodynamic and metabolic changes, and is the most serious complication related to diabetes mellitus at the level of the renal microvasculature because it leads to increased mortality and morbidity.

According to Meza, San Martm, Ruiz and Frugone its pathophysiology is not entirely clear, but the principle governing it is uncontrolled or poorly controlled hyperglycaemia accompanied by arterial hypertension, the risk factors being those already mentioned and including smoking. 44, 45, [46]

The main and worst complication it causes in advanced stages is CKD due to progressive and long-term deterioration of the kidneys. Its symptoms are noticeable in advanced stages such as the presence of protein in the urine, swelling of the lower limbs and eyelids, reduction of the amount of urine, hypertension, among others.

Although some countries do not have statistics on the subject, references are available for non-Hispanic countries, but the local data are not different from those of Europe or the United States. Incidence data provided by the United States Renal Data System (USRD) show an exponential increase: in 1996 for every million inhabitants 79,917 suffered from this disease and in 2014 for every million the sum rose to 118,014, from this data we have that 44.2% corresponded to RDD and 28.6% to hypertensive nephropaUa. The most affected age group is between 45 and 74 years in more than 60% of cases. [47, 48]

Regarding the correlation between DM and CKD, it is estimated that the risk of developing CKD is magnified; between 25-40% of patients with DM will have some degree of CKD but its prevalence will depend on other factors such as genetic predisposition, glucose and blood pressure control, smoking, among others. DM is the leading cause of chronic kidney disease worldwide, so treatment and prevention must be key points of investigation in order to provide quality healthcare and improve patients' life expectancy. [49]

The person suffering from DM generally has a higher glomerular filtration rate (GFR), due to the relaxation of the efferent arterioles, which increases the blood flow through the capillary and raises the pressure, if these conditions are maintained it causes tissue hypertrophy and, therefore, increases the capillary surface area, which translates into haemodynamic alterations that influence the development and/or progression of DRE. 50, [51]

Another of the relational factors that type 2 DM and renal diseases have in common is age, in people over 65 years of age morbidity is more than double that of younger people, this is due to the fact that there is a physiological loss of nephron function over the years, but if we add the fact of suffering from decompensated DM this will act as an inducing factor that accelerates cell death. Thus, as there is a double risk factor, old age and hyperglycaemia can trigger renal problems such as advanced kidney disease and associated pathologies such as ESRD. 52, 53, [54]

Blood pressure levels should be controlled in the person with diabetes, since increases in hydrostatic pressure at the renal glomerular level lead to glomerulosclerosis, destruction of peritubular capillaries, facilitating increased protein filtration, production of proinflammatory and profibrotic factors leading to DRE. 55, 56

Diagnosis and clinical evolution

The first clinical manifestation of DRE is the presence of albuminuria. This is an elevation of albumin excretion above the normal range.

Albuminuria in type 1 DM starts between 2 to 8 years after diagnosis of diabetes mellitus and peaks at 15 years of age. Initially albuminuria is fluctuating and there is no categorical cut-off point. At this stage there are already significant morphological alterations. In most patients albuminuria is initially reversible. When albuminuria becomes permanent, the risk of progression to proteinuria and CKD increases by 400 to 500%.

In type 2 DM, the time of onset of clinical DRD is more difficult to determine, occasionally debuting with albuminuria, proteinuria or renal failure. 57

There is consensus that in both type 1 and type 2 DM, early intervention is key to slowing the rate of progression or avoiding the onset of diabetic nephropathy altogether. This is why early detection is so important.

Albuminuria is considered to be a good predictor of clinical RDD. Its detection is not specific for DRE and it is now considered a marker of endothelial dysfunction and vascular disease, so that it is not only a predictor of nephropathy, but also of cardiovascular and overall mortality in both diabetic and non-diabetic patients.

The onset of proteinuria is not as early as is often believed; virtually all patients with microalbuminuria already have significant structural changes in renal biopsies performed by protocol, which suggests that much of the evolution of DRE takes place in clinical silence, with albumin clearance in the normal range. [58]

In the Gentofte-Montecatini convention, the presence of albuminuria was specified as the emission of albumin above 30 and up to 300 mg/day/1.73m2, with an excretion rate of 20 to 200 pg/min/1.73m2. Persistent albuminuria is present when at least two out of three determinations are positive. [59]

The determination of albuminuria is currently the first marker that exists to detect the existence of incipient renal impairment and is easy to obtain. The importance of delaying the progression of this disease can be achieved with various preventive measures: strict glycaemic control in diabetics, dietary modifications (amount of salt, proteins), compliance with pharmacological treatment, elimination of toxic habits such as smoking, treatment of hyperlipidaemia, control of arterial hypertension, etc. 60, [61]

From the above it is clear that the evolution of the person suffering from DM towards RDD is a multifactorial process that involves poor control, not only of DM as such, but also of concomitant diseases such as: arterial hypertension, obesity, previous renal diseases and/or the state of renal function, the use and misuse of medications that can alter the development of renal function and the existence or not of personal care and family support that involves eating an adequate diet, regular physical activity and maintaining adequate medical controls. 64,65

But despite all possible efforts in the field of prevention and control, according to the study by Vazquez, Cervantes, SoKs, t. al. 66 preventive interventions are insufficient and of low quality. Most of the diagnosed cases do have access to medical care, but ideally there should be an improvement in metabolic control and a lower rate of cases presenting complications in the long and medium term, this will only be possible thanks to a rethinking of the way in which care is provided by health services, to provide quality care and therefore also to provide timely diagnosis. We are clear that all these factors will act synergistically to increase or decrease the risk of developing a DRE in people with DM. 67, 68,69

Chronic Kidney Disease (CKD)

It is the progressive deterioration of renal function characterised by a decrease in the capacity of the kidney to filter blood and the consequent accumulation of nitrogenous substances in the blood, mainly urea and its derivatives, as well as creatinine, over a period of more than 3 months. [70]

CKD is a major public health problem, associated with premature mortality, with important social and economic implications. Globally, an estimated 850 million people have CKD. CKD causes at least 2.4 million deaths per year, is one of the fastest growing causes of death, and is described by nephrologists as the silent epidemic of the 21st century. It is estimated that by 2040, CKD will be the fifth leading cause of life years lost worldwide. [58, 59,70]

On the other hand, most people with CKD, especially in its early stages, are unaware of their disease, which can progress for many years without the interventions required to avoid its complications, mainly cardiovascular.

The international organisation KDIGO defines CKD as the presence of impairment of renal structure or function for a period of more than three months, with health consequences regardless of the cause as evidenced by various criteria:

> The decrease in glomerular filtration rate (GFR) < 60 mL/min/1,73 m^2

> The presence of renal injury or damage, referring to the existence of structural or functional alterations of the kidney detected directly in the renal biopsy or indirectly, by the presence of albuminuria, proteinuria, alterations in the urinary sediment, in imaging, hydroelectrolytic or other tests of tubular origin or history of renal transplantation.

It should be noted that only one of the two criteria is sufficient to diagnose CKD, and it should be stressed that the presence of renal injury markers is essential to classify a patient with CKD if the GFR is > 60 mL/min/1.73 m2.

The presence of high concentrations of prothrombin or albumin in urine is, together with GFR, the basis for the current diagnosis and staging of CKD.[72]

Currently most cases are diagnosed in advanced stages because the symptoms appear when more than 70% of kidney function has been lost. However, it is possible to detect the disease at an early stage with a simple urine test where the presence of prothrombin, a sign that kidney damage has already started, can be detected. Possible kidney damage should be suspected if there is more frequent urination in the early morning and foaming of the urine (similar to a beaten egg), and if there is weight loss or swelling in the ankles, legs and eyelids. [61-70]

If the disease is not detected at an early stage and not treated, complications such as cardiovascular disease (heart attack or stroke) can occur, which are the leading cause of death in patients with CKD before they require dialysis. Sixty percent of deaths from stroke or heart attack are in patients who already have CKD and most deaths from CKD occur before patients enter dialysis treatment.

Early detection is important, because if 10-40% of kidney function has already been lost, it is still possible to stop the progression of the disease and prevent the patient from going on dialysis- [54, 72]

Kidney diseases are silent killers that will greatly affect quality of life. However, there are several easy ways to reduce the risk of developing kidney disease, such as keeping fit, regular blood sugar checks, controlling blood pressure, eating healthy and keeping weight under control. Also, eat a healthy intake of fluids, avoid smoking and taking medications without a prescription, check kidney function if there are high risk factors (DM, HTN, overweight or a family history of kidney disease). [72, 73]

It is preventable but not curable, it is usually progressive, silent and does not present symptoms until advanced stages, when the solutions, dialysis and kidney transplantation, are already highly invasive and expensive. Many countries lack sufficient resources to purchase the necessary equipment or cover these treatments for all those who need them. Prevention for CKD in the general population is to lead a healthy lifestyle, which includes avoiding being overweight and maintaining regular physical activity, whether it be sports, walking, cycling, etc. [72]
An important part is nutrition, especially the reduction of sodium, increase of potassium intake, reduction of calories and saturated fats, among others, with a special focus on diet. Therefore, the importance of prevention, promoting healthy lifestyles, which are lifestyle modifications, such as weight control, regular exercise, sodium restriction, avoidance of alcohol, are important pillars in the treatment of a patient with DM. [73]

Risk factors affecting progression of CKD

Cardiovascular risk factors that promote the onset or affect the progression of CKD can be modifiable and non-modifiable.

<u>Non-modifiable risk factors</u>

> Genetic predisposition: Multiple genetic studies have suggested links between CKD and a variety of polymorphisms of multiple gene synthesising molecules, such as renin angiotensin aldosterone axis factors, metric oxide synthase, tumour necrosis factor alpha and multiple cytokines.

> Racial factors: These play a special role in susceptibility to CKD, reflected in the high prevalence of HTN and DM in the African-American and Afro-Caribbean populations. Socio-economic factors such as low socio-economic status have been associated with increased prevalence of CKD.

> Maternal-fetal factors Maternal undernutrition during pregnancy and excess calorie intake by the newborn may favour the development of AHT, DM, metabolic syndrome and CKD in adulthood. Low birth weight has been associated with hypertension due to a reduced number of nephrons at birth (oligonephronia), which, because of the inability to handle high solute and salt loads, leads to compensatory hypertrophy, which favours the development of glomerulosclerosis and CKD.

> Age The rate of progression of CKD is influenced by progressive increase in age.

> Sex: In univariate analyses, male gender was associated with greater deterioration of GFR, but this behaviour could not be confirmed in multivariate analyses.

<u>Modifiable risk factors</u>

Among the predictors of accelerated progression of CKD, the following have been documented in the literature as risk factors:

> **<u>Blood pressure control</u>**: Blood pressure control is a clear goal in the management of patients with CKD. Elevated systemic BP has been associated with an increase in pressure at the glomerular level, causing chronic haemodynamic alterations of the afferent arteriole and leading to a phenomenon known as adaptive hyperfiltration. This is possibly the initial phase of CKD. The most relevant haemodynamic changes in this process are:

- Compensatory response of the nephron to maintain GFR.
- Primary renal vasodilation, which occurs in patients with DM and other disorders.

It is important to emphasise that not only pathologies involving the glomerulus are important in the progression of CKD; we also find pathologies involving the tubule, causing tubular injury and accelerated progression of CKD.

> Proteinuria

Control of proteinuria is a well-established therapeutic goal in the CKD patient, as recommended by the American Heart Association. The presence of proteinuria has been considered as an independent risk factor for cardiovascular disease and progression of CKD. Multiple studies and several systematic reviews of the literature confirm the association between proteinuria and the presentation of cardiovascular events.

Proposed mechanisms of renal injury include mesangial toxicity, hyperplasia and tubular overload, direct toxicity related to compounds filtered and subsequently reabsorbed at the tubular level such as transferrin, iron and fatty acid-bound albumin. Induction of chemotactic protein binding factor 1 (MPC1) and inflammatory cytokines. The marked increase in protein filtration and proximal protein reabsorption causes tubular injury by release of lysozyme into the interstitium.

Lowering the degree of proteinuria with medication and better control of BP may decrease haemodynamic changes at the glomerular level leading to less injury and ultimately decrease the rate of renal function loss).

The search for antiproteinuric drugs has been the subject of investigation; the use of antihypertensive drugs such as antiotensin-converting enzyme inhibitors (ACE inhibitors), angiotensin receptor blockers (ARAS II), hydromethylglutaryl-CoA inhibitors, have focused the attention of clinicians and researchers in recent years. Other molecules such as thiazolidinediones and direct renin inhibitors have recently been investigated.

> **Dyslipidaemia**

It has been reported that metabolic control, hyperlipaemia and metabolic acidosis may be associated with progression of CKD. The SHARP study provided adequate evidence on the efficacy and safety of lowering LDL-cholesterol levels on the incidence of major atherosclerotic events in CKD patients without renal supportive therapy. Although a decrease in impaired GFR calculated by the MDRD4 and COCKCROFT GAULT formulas was found in patients treated with sinvastatin, no statistically significant difference was reached, however, the statin may have a renoprotective effect in those patients with CKD and cardiovascular disease.

> **Smoking**

Smoking increases blood pressure and affects renal haemodynamics. In both diabetic and non-diabetic patients, smoking is an independent factor in the progression of CKD.

> **Obesity**

Obesity has been identified in several studies as a risk factor for the development and progression of CKD.

A higher prevalence of proteinuria has been seen in the obese population, with the development of focal and segmental glomerular sclerosis as a finding in the renal histopathology of these patients. The pathophysiology is not fully understood, theories of haemodynamic changes, increased vasoactive and fibrogenic substances, including angiotensin II, insulin, leptin and transforming growth factor

beta, have been proposed.
Among the haemodynamic changes reported are phenomena of glomerular hyperfiltration in obese patients, as well as higher than average tubular sodium reabsorption in the general population.
Hyperlipaemia is a common disorder in obese patients, as are hyperglycaemia and other metabolic disorders. In multiple rodent animal models, accumulation of triglyceride and cholesterol vesfcules has been found at the level of the renal medulla. Other substances, such as plasminogen activator 1 (PAI-1), Vascular Endothelium Derived Growth Factor (VEGF), Collagen type IV and Fibronectin, are found to be elevated in obese patients.
The activation of the Renin Angiotensin Aldosterone System from visceral adipose tissue favours the elevation of plasma renin and Angiotensin II levels characteristic of these patients and which contribute to haemodynamic and renal changes. High aldosterone levels are common in the obese and these aldosterone levels are independent of renin levels, favouring more sodium reabsorption at the distal nephron. In these patients, hyperinsulinaemia favours the presence of insulin-dependent growth factors leading to the formation of glomerulosclerosis.

> **<u>Alcohol and other</u>**

Some evidence supports that alcohol consumption of more than 1.5 kquid ounces (44 ml) of alcohol (American or Scotch whisky, vodka, gin, etc.) or 4 kquid ounces (118 ml) of wine or 12 kquid ounces (355 ml) of beer per day may promote the progression of CKD.
The set of measures aimed at correcting the accelerating factors of kidney disease is what makes it possible to achieve a better quality of life in this type of patient.[73]
It is necessary for patients with DM to learn more about their disease. It is incumbent on health care providers to provide them with the means to improve their health and in turn to exercise greater control over their health. To achieve an adequate state of physical, mental and social well-being, an individual or group must be able to identify and realise their aspirations, meet their needs, change or adapt to their environment.

CHAPTER 4

METHODOLOGICAL DESIGN

A pre-experimental, prospective, intervention study was carried out to prevent CKD in type 2 diabetic patients of the family medical offices 47 and 48 of the XX Aniversario polyclinic, Santa Clara municipality, Villa Clara province, in the period between June 2022 and March 2024. The universe consisted of 177 type 2 diabetic patients belonging to the family doctor's offices and the sample consisted of 60 of them, selected with a non-probabilistic intentional sampling, who had to fulfil the inclusion criteria with prior informed consent (Annex 1).

Inclusion criteria

> Patients with a diagnosis of type 2 DM who volunteered to participate in the research through informed consent (Annex 1).

Exclusion criteria

> Type 2 diabetic patients with cognitive impairment and/or mental retardation, whether mild, moderate or severe.

> Type 2 diabetic patients previously diagnosed with CKD.

> Type 2 diabetic patients who are unable to travel to the educational activity.

Exit criteria

> Type 2 diabetic patients who will miss more than 20% of the activities that will take place.

> Type 2 diabetic patients who dropped out of the study due to circumstances such as death, long hospital stays or leaving the country for certain circumstances.

> Type 2 diabetic patients who do not wish to continue in the study.

Research methods used

The general methods of the theoretical and empirical level were used. The mathematical-statistical methods were also used.

Theoretical methods

> Historical-logical: They were used to study the history of DM and CKD in diabetic patients, their current situation at the global, national and provincial levels.

> Analysis and synthesis: This consisted in internalising the causes of the

The following table provides an overview of the topics that are not well known, as well as the topics that are less well prepared, and to draw conclusions from the literature reviewed.

> Induction and deduction: It allowed to work from the individual particularity of the patients, to logically identify their reasoning, starting from particular to general knowledge.

> System approach: This research began by recognising the system character of each component of the problem, in order not to
to look at it in isolation and be able to achieve improvements in quality of life.

Empirical methods

> Documentary analysis: A review of individual clinical histories and family records was carried out in order to describe the study sample according to clinical and epidemiological variables, which were collected on a data form (Annex 2).

> Diagnostic questionnaire: Aimed at patients with the objective of determining the level of information on CKD prevention in diabetic patients, consisting of 8 questions

in which the information they fear about the subject is specified (Annex 3).

> Observation: This was done by reviewing the results of urine tests performed to measure albuminuria as one of the markers of renal damage. The findings obtained through the researcher's observation were reflected in an observation guide (Annex 4).

> Questionnaire to specialists: Used for the assessment by the specialists of the educational actions before putting them into practice (Annex 5).

> Evaluation questionnaire: Addressed to patients with the aim of assessing their level of information after the educational actions have been applied (Annex 3).

Mathematical-statistical methods

Methods of descriptive and inferential statistics were used to represent the data in tables and texts for analysis and interpretation, based on the characteristics of the variables treated. The mathematical percentage was used. For the statistical processing of the collected data, a database was created in Excel and a SPSS file version 24.0 for Windows, with this statistical package all the collected information was processed, reflected in tables and statistical tests were carried out.

Operationalisation of variables

Variable	Classification	Description	Scale
Age	Quantitative discreet	Years of service	- 20-39 years old - 40-59 years old - 60 - 79 years old - Aged 80 and over.
Sex	Qualitative nominal dichotomous	Biological condition at birth	■ Female ■ Male
Schooling	Qualitative ordinal	Last level school approved	■ Primary ■ Secondary ■ Pre-university ■ Medium technician ■ University
Body Mass Index	Qualitative nominal polytomatic	According to the calculation of the formula BMI= current weight (kg) / height $(m)^2$	■ Underweight: Less than 18.5. ■ Normal weight: from 18,524.9 ■ Overweight. From 25.029.9. ■ Obesity. Older than
			30.
Time of evolution of the DM	Quantitative discreet	Refers to the time elapsed in years since the diagnosis was made.	■ 5 years or less ■ From 6 -10 years ■ Older than 10 years.
Risk factors for CKD,	Qualitative nominal	Refers to a certain characteristic	■ Hyperglycaemia ■ Arterial hypertension

	polytomous	present in the person that is associated with CKD.	■ Dyslipidaemia ■ Ischaemic CardiopaUa ■ Obesity ■ Smoking ■ Consumption of alcoholic beverages ■ Consumption of nephrotoxic drugs ■ Family history of renal disease ■ Other. Which
Albuminuria	Qualitative nominal	According to the presence of albumin in a sample of	■ Negative: less than 20 mg/l ■ Positive: between 20-200
	dichotomous	urine in the morning.	mg/l
Level of information of diabetic patients about risk factors that can cause CKD	Qualitative ordinal	Referred to the level of information on risk factors that can cause CKD.	■ High: if 5 or more risk factors are met ■ Medium: if between 2 and 4 risk factors respond. ■ Low: if they answer 1 or no type
Level of information of diabetic patients on the main clinical manifestations of CKD	Qualitative ordinal	Referring to the level of information on the main clinical manifestations of CKD	■ High: if you respond to 3 or more clinical manifestations ■ Medium: if 2 clinical manifestations are responded to ■ Low: if you respond 1 or no clinical manifestations
Level of information of diabetic patients about complications of CKD	Qualitative ordinal	Referring to the level of information on complications of CKD	■ High: if they respond to 5 or more complications ■ Medium: if they answer correctly between 2 and 4 complications ■ Low: if they respond 1 or no complication
Level of	Variable	Referred to the level	High: if you answer 3 or
informing diabetic patients about measures they can take to prevent CKD	qualitative nominal	of information on measures that could be taken to prevent CKD.	further measures ■ Medium: yes answer 2 measures ■ Low: if you answer 1 or

			no measure
Assessment of educational actions according to the criteria of specialists.	Nominal qualitative variable	Related to the valuation of actions designed by specialists	■ Accepted: When 86 to 100 % of the consulted specialists evaluated the requested aspects with 4 or 5 and no aspect is evaluated by the specialists with less than 3. ■ Accepted with recommendations: When between 70 and 85 % of the consulted specialists evaluated the requested aspects with 4 or 5 and no aspect was evaluated with less than 3. ■ Not Accepted: When the results are not in accordance with the above.
			defined.
Effectiveness of educational actions	Qualitative nominal dichotomous	Ratio between achieved and proposed results	■ Effective: When 85% or more of the study sample increases the level of information. ■ Not effective: When less than 85 % of the study sample achieves an increase in the level of information.

Techniques and procedures for the collection and processing of information
To begin the research, a thorough bibliographical review and an in-depth analysis of the subject was carried out, in relation to the most relevant aspects of the subject in the national and international sphere. Authorisation for the execution of this study was requested from the management of the institution involved in the development of the study and their informed consent in order to guarantee the administrative support to carry out the actions for the improvement of the quality of life of these people. The research process was carried out in four stages

First stage: Diagnosis
Patients were summoned to the clinic and, if there were any impediments, their homes were visited in order to explain the objectives of the research and to request the informed consent of the patients to participate in the research (Annex 1).
Individual medical histories and family records were reviewed and a data form was filled in by the researcher, where information related to demographic, clinical and

epidemiological variables of interest was collected (Annex 2).

All patients in the study group were tested for albuminuria as the best and earliest marker of DRE at the beginning of the study, and this information was collected in an observation guide (Annex 3). For this purpose, urine samples were collected in a sterile bottle and processed in the clinical laboratory of the XX Aniversario polyclinic.

A diagnostic questionnaire was then applied in order to identify the level of information of diabetic patients about CKD (Annex 4). The questionnaire consisted of eight questions related to essential aspects of DM and CKD. The researcher scored the questionnaire taking into account the instructions designed for the questionnaire (Annex 5).

Second stage: Design.

At this stage, initially, taking into account the results obtained in the previous stage, a document was drawn up that included the main socio-demographic characteristics of the study sample, the description of the level of information and the main difficulties diagnosed.

This document was distributed to the members of a **focus group** (Annex 6) which consisted of five specialists:

> A first-degree specialist in Internal Medicine with teaching status.

> A first degree specialist in Endocrinology with teaching status.

> One first degree specialist in Nephrology with teaching category

> A first-degree specialist in General Comprehensive Medicine with teaching status.

> An experienced psychologist and teacher.

This group was asked to hold a working session in which the topics to be worked on, related to the level of information on CKD, were raised, and the group worked on the proposed topics to be covered in the educational programme. Once the possible topics to be addressed had been defined, they were subjected to analysis by a **nominal group** (Annex 7) to reach a consensus on which aspects should form part of the design. This group was made up of five specialists:

> A first-degree specialist in Nephrology with a teaching category, lecturer-instructor.

> A first-degree specialist in Internal Medicine with teaching status.

> A first degree specialist in General Comprehensive Medicine and Master in Medical Emergencies, with teaching category, instructor professor.

> Degree in Psychology, with teaching assistant professor status.

> Degree in Pedagogy, with teaching experience, Master in Advanced Education and assistant teacher.

The group agreed on the definition of the structure, topics, teaching aids, organisational form and aspects to be evaluated to determine its effectiveness after implementation.

Subsequently, the educational programme was designed on the basis of the diagnosis carried out previously, the structure of the programme included an introduction, rationale, objectives, structural components, methodological requirements and evaluation.

Next, the **evaluation of** the designed educational programme **by specialists** (Annex 8) was taken into account, the aim of the technique was to achieve a reliable consensus among the opinions of the group of specialists, by means of a questionnaire that was answered anonymously. The sample for the evaluation of the proposed design was selected and consisted of seven specialists:

> A first degree specialist in Nephrology with more than 10 years of professional experience, lecturer and assistant professor.

> A first degree specialist in Endocrinology with more than 10 years of professional experience, lecturer and assistant professor.

> A first degree specialist in Internal Medicine with more than 10 years of professional experience, lecturer and assistant professor.

> A first degree specialist in General Comprehensive Medicine, with more than 10 years of professional and teaching experience and assistant professors.

> A second degree specialist in General Comprehensive Medicine with more than 30 years of professional and teaching experience.

> A graduate in Psychology with teaching category of teacher instructor.

> A Bachelor in Pedagogy with 25 years of teaching experience.

As indicators to be evaluated, the structure, relevance, usefulness, feasibility and scientific value were taken into account and the following evaluation categories were considered:

> Accepted: When 86 to 100 % of the consulted specialists evaluated the requested aspects with 4 or 5 and no aspect was evaluated by the specialists with less than 3.

> Accepted with recommendations: When between 70 and 85 % of the consulted specialists evaluated the requested aspects out of 4 or 5 and no aspect was evaluated with less than 3.

> Not Accepted: When the results did not conform to the above definition.

In order to carry out the assessment, the specialists had to fill in the following table on the basis of the indications given and after delivery of the designed product.

No	Aspects to Evaluate	1	2	3	4	5
1	Structure					
2	Relevance					
3	Utility					
4	Feasibility					
5	Scientific value					

The evaluative categories were explained by the researcher, the score to be given was in ascending order, the evaluation given was also qualitatively represented in the following way: 5 (excellent), 4 (good), 3 (fair) and less (poor) and it was specified that if it was less than 5 they should express below the table which aspect led them to make that decision.

The operational definitions to give the corresponding evaluation for each aspect were:

Structure: whether it was in line with actions to increase the level of information to prevent CKD in patients with type 2 DM.

Relevance: whether the way in which the actions were conceived responded to the difficulties identified in the diagnosis.

Utility: if the designed product responds to an identified and unresolved problem.

Feasibility: whether the actions could be implemented in practice.

Scientific value: if the results obtained were the result of scientific research, carried out through a rigorous research process and the detection of risk factors for CKD.

Third stage: Implementation.

After the necessary conditions were established, the educational programme was implemented (Annex 9). The participants were divided into two groups of 30 people each and the programme was delivered in two stages: an intensive first stage and a second reinforcement stage. The intensive stage lasted three months and was delivered in five weeks, every fortnight for each subgroup, each lasting one hour. The reinforcement stage was carried out in three months with a monthly frequency for each subgroup with a duration of one hour each. In the last month, the two subgroups were unified to carry out the final activity. The activities were carried out in the primary school 28 de Enero, within the radius of action of the clinic, which facilitated the accessibility of the participants to the activities and had as responsible the author of the research and the family doctor of these clinics who contributed with the organisation of each one of the activities.

Stage 4: Evaluation.

Once the educational actions were concluded, in the last meeting, an evaluation questionnaire was applied to the participants (Annex 4). The same evaluation parameters were considered as in the diagnostic stage.

For the determination of the effectiveness of the educational programme, 85 % or more of the study sample reached an adequate level of information about CKD. and the application of hypothesis tests to determine the significance of the favourable changes that occurred, in relation to the high level of information of type 2 diabetic patients about CKD risk factors.

Statistical processing of data

Data processing was carried out on a microcomputer with a Windows 10 operating system. The data were processed using the statistical programme SPSS version 26.0, descriptive statistics, using absolute numbers and percentage calculation for the total of the variables, and inferential statistics (hypothesis test of proportions with a value for $p<0.05$). The results were presented in the form of texts and statistical tables of frequency distribution, using Microsoft Office software.

Ethical considerations

This study was conducted in accordance with the ethical principles for medical research involving human subjects set out in the Declaration of Helsinki. The patients included in the research were voluntary participants whose consent was requested in order to obtain their willingness and cooperation in the research performance, respecting at all times the refusal to participate (Annex 1). The results of this study will only be used for scientific purposes and the author undertook not to disclose data that could be used to identify the members of the sample.

CHAPTER 5

ANALYSIS AND DISCUSSION OF THE RESULTS

DM is one of the main risk factors for CKD, so it is necessary for every patient suffering from the disease to be able to control and prevent the progression of the disease towards CKD through their own actions.

Table I.Distribution of patients with type 2 diabetes mellitus according to age and sex.

Age groups (years)	Female		Male		Total	
	No.	%	No.	%	No.	%
20 - 39	7	11,7	2	3.3	9	15.0
40 - 59	6	10.0	9	15.0	15	25.0
60 - 79	21	40.4	11	21.1	32	53.3
80 and over	2	3.33	2	3.8	4	6.7
Total	41	68.3	19	321.7	60	100.0

Source: Data form

Table 1 shows the distribution of the type 2 diabetic patients who participated in the study according to age and sex. Female patients predominated with 68.3 %.

According to the author, this may be due to the taboos that still exist among the male sex that it is women who should participate in this type of activity, as well as the fact that men are more involved in working life than women, which sometimes makes it difficult for them to participate in this type of study.

This also coincides with studies, such as that of Toala, Rosa and others, which show that DM occurs more frequently among the female sex. [74, 75, 76]

This is at odds with the results found in other studies such as that of Russo[77] and the International Diabetes Federation (IDF) 78, which state that with regard to biological sex, a higher prevalence is estimated in men compared to women.

In relation to the age group that predominated in the study, this was the group between 60 and 79 years of age, representing 53.3 %. According to the author, these results may be due to the fact that statistically it is in the older age groups where the highest prevalence of the disease has been shown to be found.

It can be added that this stage of life coincides with the retirement stage of working life, which means that there is more time available to participate in this type of educational activities.

This study is consistent with Avila Gonzalez's findings on the increase in the diagnosis of DM with increasing age, with more than a quarter of the world's population aged 60-69 years predominating. [79]

This average age in adults with MD is relevant, as it reinforces it as a health problem that needs to be addressed in a complex phenomenon, such as all the care that should be related to this disease. [77, 78, 80]

Table 2. Distribution of type 2 diabetic patients by level of education

Level of schooling	No.	%
Unfinished primary school	3	5.0
Completed primary school	6	10.0

Secondary	15	25.0
Pre-university	26	43.3
University	10	16.7
Total	60	100.0

Source: Data form

Table 2 shows the level of education of the type 2 diabetic patients who participated in the study, showing a predominance of pre-university level with 43.3 % followed by secondary level with 25 %.

According to the author, the level of education is an important factor for the control of DM, as well as for the prevention of CKD, because as the level of education increases, patients become more interested in their disease and the measures to control it and avoid complications.

Likewise, those with lower levels of education are less likely to attend hospital services, have less adherence to treatment and have a lower risk perception of the consequences of treatment.

In order to ensure that patients acquire a level of information about the subject matter of the educational programme under investigation, it should be borne in mind that those with a higher level of education are more likely to reach and assimilate a greater amount of information.

This coincides with the study by Hernandez-Zambrano et al. in relation to the level of schooling, finding greater adherence to treatment and greater control of DM in people with middle and upper-middle schooling. [82]

Borroto in his study of educational intervention to modify levels of knowledge about CKD in diabetic patients, in relation to the level of schooling reflects that the highest percentage is at the pre-university level, followed by those at university level, concluding that the higher the level of schooling, the higher the level of knowledge. [83]

Table 3. Distribution of type 2 diabetic patients according to body mass index.

BMI	No.	%
Underweight	5	8.3
Normopeso	18	30.0
Overweight	24	40.0
Obese	13	21.7
Total	60	100.0

Source: Data form

Table 3 shows the behaviour of the body mass index (BMI) of the type 2 diabetic patients who participated in the study, showing that there was a predominance of overweight patients with 40 %, followed by normal weight patients with 30 %, and not less important, in third place were the obese patients who represented 21.7 % of the total.

Body mass index is a frequently used indicator to identify overweight and obesity in adults. A high body mass index is one of the most important risk factors for the development of CKD.

According to the author, although it was not obesity that came first in the study, it was worrying that at least part of the study sample presented this condition, so it was necessary to try to raise the level of information of patients to reverse this condition, in addition to the fact that overweight patients predominated, and educational activity took value to try to prevent them from becoming obese and thus reduce the occurrence of CKD.

Mohammedi in his study on the association of body mass index and the risk of renal events in patients with type 2 DM points out that high BMI is a predictor of renal events in patients with type 2 DM and that weight loss is an important strategy to achieve nephroprotection of diabetic patients. [84]

Table 4. Distribution of type 2 diabetic patients according to risk factors for CKD

Risk factors	No.	%
Arterial hypertension	44	73.3
Dyslipidaemia	51	85.0
Ischaemic CardiopaUa	11	18.3
Obesity	13	21.7
Smoking	19	31.7
Consumption of alcoholic beverages	9	15.0
Consumption of nephrotoxic drugs	7	11.6
Family history of renal disease	8	15.3

Source: Data formn=60

The risk of developing DRE will be directly related to the number of risk factors the patient presents and the care the patient provides for each of them to keep them under control.

Table 4 shows the distribution of the type 2 diabetic patients who participated in the study according to risk factors for developing CKD. It shows that there was a predominance of dyslipidaemia (85 %), followed by hypertension and smoking (73.3 % and 31.7 % respectively).

Similar results have been reported in international studies such as those of Polanco-Flores,[85] Gheith,[86] and others,[87, 88] , with the main risk factors associated with CKD being a family history of ESRD, hypertension, dyslipidaemia and smoking.

The results obtained in this research confirm and coincide with those presented by other authors, who consider dyslipidaemia to be an important risk factor related to the development of CKD. [89, 90, 91]

Tziomalos in his study has found an association between dyslipidaemia and the occurrence of albuminuria and a doubling of serum creatinine concentrations. [92]

Elevated blood pressure in diabetic patients has been shown to increase the risk of developing RDD. [92, 93] Results found in a meta-analysis study by Wagnew that included 27 studies from several sub-Saharan African countries found that diabetics with high blood pressure had a 1.67 times higher risk of DRD than patients without high blood pressure. [94]

Smoking has been linked to the incidence of CKD. It is a recognised risk factor as an independent renal risk factor, although its mechanisms are not established.

It must be considered one of the most important remediable risk factors, therefore abstinence from smoking is a priority recommendation in CKD.

Some studies have shown that smoking almost doubled the risk of CKD in the participating subjects. [95, 96]

In a meta-analysis, the risk of developing CKD was 1.27 for ever smokers, 1.34 for

current smokers and 1.15 for former smokers compared to never smokers. [97]
Several studies have investigated the association between alcohol consumption and CKD risk and have revealed inconsistent results. A recent systematic review and dose-response meta-analysis found that light alcohol consumption (24 g/day) is protective against CKD in adult participants, especially in men. [98]
With respect to familial factors, siblings of patients with RDD have been reported to have a fivefold increased risk of the condition[92, 99] and a genome-based statistical predictive model has recently been constructed that estimates the genetic risk of RDD.
This prediction model allows to confirm the importance of the Genetic Risk Score combined with clinical factors in the prediction and identification of individuals at high risk of DRD for timely medical intervention.[100]
The author considers that many of the risk factors that are present are modifiable, such as dyslipidaemia, smoking, alcoholism, obesity and the use of nephrotoxic drugs.
Hence the importance of providing patients with the necessary information so that they themselves can modify these factors, and those that cannot be modified, at least be controlled to avoid developing CKD.
Table 5. Distribution of type 2 diabetic patients according to albuminuria and time of progression of DM.

Time of evolution (years)	**Albuminuria**					
	Negative		**Positive**		**Total**	
	No.	%	No.	%	No.	%
5 years or less	12	20.0	6	10.0	18	30.0
From 6 to 10	10	16,7	19	31.6	29	48.3
Major of 10	3	5.0	10	16.7	13	21.7
Total	25	41.7	35	58.3	60	100.0

Source: Data form and observation guide

Table 5 shows the distribution of the type 2 diabetic patients who participated in the study, according to the presence or absence of albuminuria in relation to the time since diagnosis.
It was found that 58.3 % of the patients had positive albuminuria and that 48.3 % of the sample were in the group with between 6 and 10 years of evolution of the disease since its diagnosis. The relationship between the time of evolution of type 2 DM and the presence of albuminuria was evident, as albuminuria predominated in those patients with more than 6 years of evolution of the baseline disease.
According to the author, DRE is considered one of the most severe complications in patients with type 2 DM and one of the leading causes of CKD.
It is estimated that 20-40% of people with DM will show some degree of DRE during the course of their disease and one of the earliest indicators of DRE is albuminuria, which is small amounts of albumin present in the urine and which becomes more frequent as the time since diagnosis of type 2 DM increases.
In the literature, there is controversy about the association of duration of DM as a

predictor of DRD. Hung in a cohort study with a median follow-up of 2.9 years found that patients with more than 8 years of DM duration relative to those with less than 8 years of disease were at higher risk of CKD. [101]
Liang et al. show that duration of DM is the strongest predictor of DRE in multivariate analysis, and that duration greater than 8 years is the optimal cut-off point for predicting DRE. [102, 103,104]
However, Mazzucco finds no difference in the duration of DM and DRD and non-diabetic disease. Considering that diabetic disease develops several years prior to diagnosis, the known duration of DM would not be an accurate and reliable predictor of ERD. [105]
Currently, early detection of albuminuria in patients with type 2 DM is considered to be the best and earliest marker of DRE.
Because of the importance of this marker of renal damage and its consequences, it is necessary to educate diabetic patients to provide them with all the information related to the subject so that they can adopt a healthy lifestyle and make changes to prevent, control or reverse albuminuria in order to preserve renal health.
Once the instruments had been applied, **methodological triangulation** was carried out, a tool that facilitated the articulation and validation of data through the cross-referencing of the information collected from the documentary analysis, the observation guide and the questionnaire, which allowed us to contrast the results in relation to the socio-demographic characteristics of the type 2 diabetic patients under study, albuminuria as an early marker of renal damage, the level of information for preventing CKD and educational diagnosis, where a low level of information related to general aspects and the prevention of CKD in patients with type 2 DM was determined.
With the results of the methodological triangulation, the diagnosis was concluded and the stage of designing the educational programme began with the presentation of the results of the diagnosis to the **focus group**, who with the application of the rain technique provided opinions for the design of the programme:
> As topics to be addressed in the programme, the following were proposed: General information on DM and RD, risk factors, main clinical manifestations and complications of CKD in type 2 diabetic patients, as well as measures to prevent it, the importance of determining albuminuria as a marker of renal damage.
> Use of educational techniques as a means of teaching (group discussion, group reflections and collective debate) and of the workshop as an organisational form.
> Development of the evaluation through the PNI (positive, negative, interesting) to know the opinion of the group on the actions carried out and the practice with teaching aids.
> For the determination of the effectiveness of the programme, the information level category was proposed to prevent CKD in patients with type 2 DM.
> Efficacy took into account that 85% or more of the study sample achieved a high level of information to prevent CKD in patients with type 2 DM.
> Encourage the active participation of diabetic patients in the intervention, for the acquisition of information about CKD in patients with type 2 DM.
> The sessions would last approximately 1 hour each, twice a week in the intensive stage for three months and once a month in the reinforcement stage, for three

months, in order to maintain motivation for the activity.

These ideas were presented to the group of professionals who made up the **nominal group**, who reached consensus on the following proposals for the design of the programme:

> That CKD constituted a health problem and was therefore of great importance for the health of the population.
importance of their knowledge and prevention.

> That the level of patient information was still insufficient.
diabetics to prevent CKD.

> That an intervention was needed in diabetic patients through an educational programme to raise the level of information to prevent CKD in patients with type 2 DM.

> That it should include actions to modify the level of information to prevent CKD in patients with type 2 DM.

The results of the focus and focus group were taken into account in the **design of the educational programme** (Annex 9).

The educational programme was structured as follows:

General aspects: Structured to be carried out in two stages, an intensive stage and a reinforcement stage. The intensive stage, conceived to be developed in three months, distributed in five sessions, with a fortnightly frequency of one hour of duration each, projected as a space for group reflection organised by the researcher. Aimed at the 60 diabetic patients selected to participate in the research and was carried out in the 28 de Enero primary school, which is located within the radius of action of the family medical offices involved in the study, in the period between June and August 2023, as part of the educational diagnosis, the cognitive deficiencies were identified and thus the need to expand different topics that contributed to enriching the level of information to prevent CKD in patients with type 2 DM was identified.

The reinforcement phase was carried out for three months in the period between September and November 2023 with the participation of the type 2 diabetic patients included in the study. In the last month the evaluation of the programme was carried out.

Title: Protecting my health

General Objective

Raise awareness among patients with type 2 DM to prevent CKD.

Structure and topics to be taught

The programme was carried out in two stages, the first intensive stage and a second reinforcement stage. The intensive stage lasted three months (June-August 2023), five activities were developed with a fortnightly frequency of one hour of duration each, developed as a space for group reflection organised by the researcher. Until the fifth session, the different planned themes were addressed based on the consensus of the focal group, the nominal group and the evaluation of the specialists. The reinforcement stage took place during three consecutive months (September-November 2023), lasting one hour, with the participation of the type 2 diabetic patients included in the study, and was carried out in the 28 de Enero primary school. In the last session the evaluation was carried out (November 2023) by applying the evaluation questionnaire (Annex 4).

Table 1. Proposed topics of the educational programme on the prevention of chronic kidney disease (CKD) in type 2 diabetic patients.

Title: "**Protecting my health**".

Intensive stage			
Theme	**Target**	**Content**	**Actions**
Session 1 "Knowing my illness".	Objectives -Create a state favourablefrom the	Presentation of the educational activity to be developed.	Constitutionde the groupsand determination of the standardsand
Theme 1 Introduction at Protecting Health" educational programme. my General information on DM	diabetic patients that facilitates group cohesion and reflection facilitating a environment suitablethat allow develop the issues to be addressed in as far as DM is concerned. -Define it methodolog^aa continue. -Motivaral group to raise interest in the issues to be addressed in relation to DM. Establish general group norms and rules. Know them DM in general	General information on the DM. Concept. Symptoms. Complications. Control illness.	rules general of the group. Exposition of the characteristics of the intervention. Expositiondel content thematic. (group reflection and collective discussion) Motivationfor the activities proposals.
Session 2 "^How I can get sick? " Topic 2: CKD. General.	-To know what is the ERC and surelation with the DM. -Explain the risk factors that risk	-ERC. Concept. General overview of the disease. Non-modifiable risk factors that can lead to CKD	Expositiondel content thematic. (group reflection and collective discussion)

Factors from	factorsthat can cause CKD in patients with DM	at the patients	Motivationfor the activities
riskthat can cause ERC at on diabetic patients.	type 2.	diabetics. -Modifiable risk factors that can cause CKD in the patients diabetics.	proposals.
Session 3 "^That I can feel?" Theme3 : Main clinical manifestations occurring in CKD	Identify them main clinical manifestations that are presented at the ERC.	ERC. Main clinical manifestations.	Exhibition at thematic content. Group reflection Collective debate
Session 4 "Recognising the danger " Theme 4: Complications that presented at the ERC.	Explain complications that can occur after the occurrence of CKD.	ERC. Main complications	Exhibition at thematic content. Group reflection Collective debate
Session 5 "I am I prepare to improve my health".	To set out the preventive measures for the occurrence of the ERC.	ERC. Main measures to prevent their occurrence.	Exhibition at thematic content. Group reflection
Theme5 : Measures for prevent CKD.			Collective debate
Reinforcement stage			
First month: General information on DM and CKD. Factors of risk that can cause cause ERC at on diabetic patients. Main clinical manifestations occurring in CKD	To assess the level of information on CKD acquired by the patients. patients diabetics participating in the educational programme.	General information on DM and CKD. Risk factors that may cause CKD at at diabetic patients. Main clinical manifestations presented at the ERC.	Expositiondel thematic content. Group reflection Collective debate

Second month: Complications that presented in the ERC. Measures to prevent it.	To assess the level of information on CKD acquired by the patients. patients diabetics participating in the educational programme	Complications that occur in CKD. Measures to prevent it.	Expositiondel thematic content. Group reflection Collective debate
Third month: The third month: It is carried out evaluationde the patients diabetic participants of the	To assess the level of information on CKD acquired by the patients. patients diabetics participating in the	Reaffirmation of the theoretical contents and acquired skills. Closure and evaluation.	Collective debate. Implementation of evaluative questionnaire. Closing and farewell
study.	educational programme		of the activity education.

Methodological requirements

Different active pedagogical techniques were used such as exposition, exposition plus discussion, debates and videos with discussion and educational actions that lead to change in unhealthy lifestyles.

Before starting the intervention and applying the educational programme, the questionnaire (Annex 4) was used to obtain an individual diagnosis of learning needs. The educational programme consisted of sessions that were developed in the form of a workshop, the evaluation of the process was participatory as an active subject, by means of self-evaluation procedures in each activity. At the end of the reinforcement stage, a final evaluation was carried out to assess the changes by applying the same instrument used at the beginning of the research (Annex 4). The evaluation of the educational programme was carried out from the perspective of finding out whether the proposed objectives were achieved and to determine whether the educational programme was beneficial.

Teaching aids: slides, videos, folders, models, and PowerPoint presentations designed for each activity.

Evaluation

Participatory techniques were applied that allowed for self-evaluation, which favoured the modification of the information level of the diabetic patients involved in the study.

The design of the educational programme was subjected to an evaluation by specialists and the following results were obtained.

Result of the evaluation of the educational programme by a specialist.

The seven specialists who formed the group for the evaluation of the structure, relevance, usefulness, feasibility and scientific value of the educational programme, once they had issued their criteria, the following results were obtained:

Aspects to Evaluate	1	2	3	4	5	6	7	Total
Structure	5	5	5	5	4	5	5	6-85,71 % acceptable 1-14 ,28 % accepted

								with recommendations
Relevance	3	5	5	5	4	4	5	7-100 % acceptable
Utility	4	5	5	5	5	5	4	7-100 % acceptable
Feasibility	5	4	5	4	5	5	4	7-100 % acceptable
Scientific value	5	4	5	5	5	5	5	7-100 % acceptable

The specialists stated that the programme was in line with actions to increase the level of information about CKD prevention in type 2 diabetic patients. After the evaluation it was found that 100 % of the specialists considered the proposal to be appropriate.

100 % of the specialists stated that the methodologies, techniques, as well as the themes responded to the objectives, while only 85.71 % considered the structure to be acceptable.

We then went on to establish the relationship between the educational programme and the level of information of the diabetic patients who participated in the programme.

Table 6: Distribution of diabetic patients according to level of information about CKD before and after the educational intervention.

Level of Information	Formerly						Then					
	High		Medium		Under		High		Medium		Under	
	No	%	No	%	No	%	No	%	No	%	No	%
Risk factors	14	23	19	32	27	45	54	90	6	10	0	0
Manifestations clmicas	19	32	20	23	21	35	54	90	8	10	0	0
Complications	17	28	19	32	24	40	56	93	4	7	0	0
Preventive measures	12	20	23	38	25	42	58	97	2	3	0	0

Source: Diagnostic and evaluative questionnaire=60

Table 6 shows the distribution of diabetic patients according to the level of information on CKD before and after the educational intervention.

It shows that before the implementation of the educational programme, diabetic patients with a low level of information on risk factors, clinical manifestations, complications and preventive measures to avoid the disease predominated, accounting for 45 %, 40 %, 35 % and 42 % respectively, followed by those with a medium level of information in each case.

It is noteworthy that in all cases less than 20% of those involved in the study had a high level of CKD-related information.

It can be seen that after the intervention, in general, an improvement was observed in the level of information about CKD acquired by diabetic patients in all cases, with no patient presenting a low level of information related to the disease and a high level of information predominating in more than 90 % of cases.

According to the author, the level of information about CKD acts as a protective factor in patients with DM, and the results obtained show the important role that can be played by comprehensive health education with special attention to prevention,

education and support.
The level of information about the characteristics of CKD causes a series of changes that significantly affect the patient's life by slowing down the progression of this chronic non-communicable disease. A simple educational intervention can improve the level of information about CKD in the population most susceptible to the disease.
The data addressed by the study coincide with some of the results of similar studies.[86] Such is the case of Garces and Dayly[106] that before the educational intervention the level of insufficient knowledge was 57 % (30 patients) and after the educational intervention it reached up to 77 %, in the same number of patients, with a sufficient level of knowledge.
Burgos Jimenez and collaborators[107] in the research work on the impact of an intervention aimed at increasing knowledge of kidney disease on the timely initiation of renal replacement therapy, highlight that in relation to knowledge of the four dimensions measured by the questionnaire, a 75.4% increase in the good level was achieved in more than 21 females who answered correctly; changes that are consistent with what has been published on the knowledge of the disease in diabetic patients.
The article referring to the level of knowledge about CKD in patients, relatives and nursing staff is also related to this study, as it identifies that in relation to patients, those with a low level (70.51 %) predominate, followed by those with a medium level (26.92 %) and only 2 patients (2.57 %) reach a high level in relation to the answers given to the research questionnaire.[108]
There is a difference with respect to Valverde and Zari[109] from Ecuador, who in their research obtained the result that the patients participating in the study had a high level of knowledge before applying the educational intervention, which does not coincide with this research, showing that most of the patients had a poor level of information.
The results obtained once the educational activity was applied, showed the increase in the level of information of type 2 diabetic patients who participated in the study to prevent CKD, **demonstrating the effectiveness of the educational programme,** as more than 90 % of diabetic patients managed to reach a high level of information. This demonstrates the importance of educating patients in the knowledge of their disease in order to facilitate the prevention of possible complications that may develop in the course of their evolution.
These results are similar to those found in the study by Garces and Dayly[106] whose population was 115, who demonstrate that the educational intervention is effective in increasing knowledge, since in the initial evaluation, 40% had a low level of knowledge with regard to self-care and it is evident that after the implementation of the educational intervention, the level of knowledge increases with 78%.
This coincides with Nola Pender's theory, which states that knowledge increases through interaction, so that people adopt behaviours that lead to an improvement in their quality of life; in other words, providing information helps to generate positive attitudes and in this way, they become aware and modify their lifestyles, reducing morbimortality in the face of a public health problem that affects a large part of the population due to a lack of knowledge.
Other similar studies reflect results that corroborate ours by demonstrating the

effectiveness in each of them after applying different types of educational activities in raising the level of information related to CKD and its prevention. [110, 111, 112,]

Other authors have shown, through the evaluation of educational and care programmes for diabetic patients, that education undoubtedly leads to better control of DM, delaying or preventing the development of complications such as CKD. [113, 114, 115]

In Sanchez's words, "Health education is a tool that allows people to take an active role in modifying their behaviours to promote health by incorporating the knowledge that can come from health professionals".

CONCLUSIONS

In this investigation, diabetic patients between 60 and 79 years of age, female sex, pre-university education and overweight prevailed. Dyslipidaemia, hypertension and smoking were the main risk factors for developing chronic kidney disease. Albuminuria was identified as an early marker of renal damage, being positive in more than 50 % of the cases and more frequent in diabetic patients with 6 or more years of evolution. Before the educational intervention, a low level of information on chronic kidney disease predominated in the sample studied, and once the educational programme was implemented, it increased in more than 90 % of cases. The educational programme: "**Protecting my health**" proved to be effective in raising the level of information of type 2 diabetic patients about CKD.

RECOMMENDATIONS

✓ Generalise the application of the educational programme in other health areas to contribute to the prevention of chronic kidney disease in type 2 diabetic patients.

✓ Continue to conduct intervention studies in PHC with the aim of improving the means of communication on the prevention of chronic kidney disease in diabetic patients.

✓ To continue the study, not only to modify the level of information on the subject, but also to try to modify the behaviour of diabetic patients in order to prevent chronic kidney disease.

BIBLIOGRAPHICAL REFERENCES

1. Ruz A, Arranz E, Garrta JC, Garrta ME, Palacios D, Montero A, et al. Prevalence of diabetes mellitus in the Spanish primary care setting and its association with cardiovascular risk factors and cardiovascular disease. SIMETAP-DM study. Clin Invest Arterioscl [Internet]. 2020 [cited 2024 my 26]; 32(1): [approx. 11p]. Available at: https://doi.org/10.1016/j.arteri.2019.03.006

2. Pavon-Rojas AJ, Escalona-Gonzalez SO, Cisnero-Reyes L, Gonzalez-Milan ZC. Microalbuminuria: a method for early detection of chronic kidney disease in diabetics. SPIMED [Internet]. 2020 [cited 5 Jun 2024]; 1(2). Available from: https://revspimed.sld.cu/index.php/spimed/article/view/15

3. Zavala-Calahorrano AM, Fernandez E. Diabetes mellitus type II in Ecuador: epidemiological review. 2018 [Thesis]. Ecuador: Universidad Tecnica de Ambato, Tungurahua; 2018. Available in: DOI: https:ZZdoi.org/10.31243/mdc.uta.v2i4.132.2018

4. International Diabetes Federation. IDF Diabetes Atlas [Internet]. 8ed. Brussels, Belgium: International Diabetes Federation; 2017 [cited 2024 my 26]. Available from: http://diabetesatlas.org/resources/2017-atlas.html

5. Ayala-Reynoso PP. Therapeutic intervention to achieve glycaemic control in patients with diabetes mellitus. [Postgraduate thesis]. Ecuador: Escuela Superior Politecnica de Chimborazo, Riobamba, Chimborazo; 2019. Available at: http://dspace.espoch.edu.ec/handle/123456789/12503

6. Kovesdy CP. Epidemiology of chronic kidney disease: anupdate 2022. Kidney Int Suppl [Internet] Apr 2022 [cited 2024 my 26]; 12(1):7-11. Available at: https://www.ncbi.nlm.nih.gov/pmc/articles/PMC9073222/

7. Polanco-Flores NA, Rodriguez-Castellanos F. Early detection of diabetic nephropaUa, about its screening. Rev Nefrol Dial Traspl [Internet] 2018 [cited 2024 my 26]; 38(4):258-67.Available from: https://www.revistarenal.org.ar/index.php/rndt/article/view/372/553

8. Turkmen K. Inflammation, oxidative stress, apoptosis, and autophagy in diabetes mellitusand diabetickidneydisease: theFourHorsemen of theApocalypse. Int Urol Nephro [Inernet]. May 2017 [cited 2024 my 26];49(5):837-44.Available from: https://pubmed.ncbi.nlm.nih.gov/28035619/

9. Sosa N, Polo RA, Mendez SN, Sosa M. Characterization of patients with chronic kidney disease on haemodialysis treatment. Medisur [Internet]. 2016 [cited 2024 my 26]; 14(4): [approx. 10p.]. Available from: http://medisur.sld.cu/index.php/medisur/article/vi ew/2969\.

10. Hernando-Avendano L. History of Nephrology in Spain. Barcelona: Ediciones Pulso; 2017. Historical background. First notes on renal diseases. p. 19 - 20

11. Cusumano AM, Rosa-Diez G. Notes for the history of dialysis in the world and in Argentina. Second part: the beginnings of haemodialysis in Argentina. Rev Nefrol Dial Traspl [Internet]. 2020 [cited 2024 my 26]; 40(3): 242-250 . Available from: https://www.revistarenal.org.ar/index.php/rndt/article/view/538

12. Herrera-Anazco P, Pacheco-Mendoza J, Taype-Rondan A. Chronic kidney disease in Peru. A narrative review of published scientific articles. Acta Med Peru

[Internet]. 2016 [cited 2024 my 26]; 33(2): 130 - 137
http://www.scielo.org.pe/pdf/amp/v33n2/a07v33n2.pdf
http://www.scielo.org.pe/pdf/amp/v33n2/a07v33n2.pdf.

13. D^az-Armas MT, Gomez-Leyva B, Robalino-Valdivieso MP, Lucero-Proano SA. Epidemiological behaviour in patients with end-stage renal disease in Ecuador. CCM [internet]. 2018 [cited 2024 my 26] (2): 312 - 324. Available from: http://scielo.sld.cu/pdf/ccm/v22n2/ccm11218.pdf

14. Lacomba-Trejo L, Mateu-Molla J, Carbajo-Alvarez E, Oltra-Benavent AM, Galan-Serrano A. Advanced chronic kidney disease. Association between anxiety, depression and resilience. Colombian Rev. Nefrol [Internet]. 2019 [cited 2024 my 26]; 6(2): 103-111 . Available from: https://revistanefrologia.org/index.php/rcn/article/view/344/pdf

15. Ram^ez-Perdomo CA, Solano-Ruiz MC. The social construction of the experience of living with chronic kidney disease. Rev. Latino-Am Enfermagen [Internet] 2028 [cited 2024 my 26]; 26: e3028. Disponible en: https://www.scielo.br/pdf/rlae/v26/es_0104-1169-rlae-26-e3028.pdf; http://dx.doi.org/10.1590/1518-8345.2439.3028

16. Gorostidi M, Santamaria R, Alcazar R, Fernandez Fresnedo G, Galceran JM, Goicoechea M, et al. Spanish Society of Nephrology document on the KDIGO guidelines for the evaluation and treatment of chronic kidney disease. Nefrolog^a [internet]. 2017 [cited2024 my 26]; 34(3): 302-316 . Available In: http://scielo.isciii.es/pdf/nefrologia/v34n3/especial2.pdf

17. Martmez Perez Denia, Perez de Alejo Rodriguez Lutgarda, More Chang Carmen Xiomara, Rodriguez Viera Ricardo, Dupuy Nunez Juan Carlos. Clinical laboratory studies for the detection of chronic kidney disease in at-risk population groups. MEDISAN [Internet]. 2016 Jan [cited 2024 Jun 05]; 20(1): 49-58. Available from: http://scielo.sld.cu/scielo.php?script=sci arttext&pid=S1029-30192016000100008&lng=es

18. Lorenzo CMB, Ortega GEA, Ortega HA, Ferreiro GLR, Carballea BM. Development of chronic kidney disease in patients with arterial hypertension and/or diabetes mellitus. Universidad Medica Pinarena [Internet]. 2019 [cited 2024 my 26]; 15(1):[approx. 10p]. Available from: https://www.medigraphic.com/cgi-bin/new/resum

19. Miranda JJ, Aleman B, Vega J, Gartia D, Arocha Y, Rivero L. Factors of progression of renal dysfunction in diabetics admitted to Internal Medicine. Rev Med Electron [Internet]. 2016 [cited 2024 my 26]; 38(6):[approx. 5p]. Available In: https://www.revmedicaelectronica.sld.cu/index.p hp/rme/article/view/1610/3207

20. Besse-Diaz R, Martmez-Cantillo L, Rfos-Vega L. Clinical and epidemiological aspects related to microalbuminuria in patients with type 2 diabetes mellitus. MEDISAN [Internet]. 2018 on [cited 2024 March 31]; 22(1): 11-18. Available In: http://scielo.sld.cu/scielo.php?script=sci arttext&pid=S1029-30192018000100002&lng=es.

21. Martell-Marthez M, Cisnero-Causillo,C, Gonzalez-Aguero J E, Galiano- Silva G. Microalbuminuria as a marker of kidneydamage in patientswith diabetes mellitus. J Clin Med Rev 2022; 1(1); 12.

22. Lin YC, Chang YH, Yang SY, Wu KD, Chu TS. Update of pathophysiology and management of diabetickidneydisease. J Formos Med Assoc Taiwan YiZhi. Aug 2018; 117(8):662-75.
23. Moreno F, Castillo C, Pena JK. Renal involvement in diabetes mellitus. Medicine [Internet]. 2019 [cited 2024 my 26]; 12(80):[approx. 9p]. Available at: https://www. medicineonline.es/en- affectacion-ren al-diabetes- mellitus-articulo-S030454121930145 3
24. Cuba. Ministry of Public Health. Anuario Estad^stico de Salud 2020 [Internet]. Havana: Direccion Nacional de Estad^sticas; 2021 [cited 2024my26]. Available from: https://files.sld.cu/bvscuba/files/2020/05/AnuarioElectronico-Espanol-2019- ed-2
25. Velez L, Fuentes M, Morieira M, Lucio L. Vulnerability to type 2 diabetes mellitus. Rev CienUfica Multidiscip. 2020; 4(3):93 - 8.
26. Lopez-Casanova A, Triana de la Paz R, Ruiz-Triana A, D^az-Alfonso NI, Gutierrez- Escarras Y. Metabolic syndrome in type 2 diabetic patients. Acta Med Cent [Internet]. 2019 [cited 2024 my 26]; 13(3):284-96. Available at: https://www.medigraphic.com/pdfs/medicadelcentro/mec-2019/mec193a.pdf
27. Altamirano L, Vasquez M, Cordero G, Alvares R, Anez R, Rojas J, et al. Prevalence of type 2 diabetes mellitus and its risk factors in adult individuals in the city of Cuenca- Ecuador. Av in Biomed [Internet]. 2017 [cited 2024 my 26]; 6(1):10-21. Available from: http://www.redalyc.org/pdf/3313/331351068003.pdf
Martmez B, Mendez Y, Veldez I. Risk factors associated with type 2 diabetes mellitus. Policlfnico Docente Jose Jacinto Milanes. Matanzas, 2019. Rev Med Electron [Internet]. 2021 [cited 2024 my 26]; 43(6):1 -13. Available from: http:/www.revmedicaelectronica.sld.cu/index.php/rme/article/view/4140/pdf:
28. Blanco-Naranjo EG, Chavarria-Campos GF, Garita-Fallas YM. Healthy lifestyle in type 2 diabetes mellitus: benefits in chronic management. Rev Medica Sinerg. 2021; 6(2):e639.
29. Peinado-Martmez M, Dager-Vergara I, Quintero-Molano K, Mogollon-Perez M, Puello-Ospina A. Metabolic syndrome in adults: a narrative review of the literature. Arch Med [Internet] 2021[cited 2024 my 26];17 (2:4) : 1-5.Available at: https://www.archivosdemedicina.com/medicina-de-family/siacutendrome-metaboacutelic-metaboacutelic-in-adults-review-narrative-of-literature.pdf
30. Perez- Gonzalez M. Metabolic syndrome in patients with type 2 diabetes mellitus. Rev Ciencias Medicas Pinar del Rfo [Internet]. 2016 [cited 2024my26]; 20(4):26-36. Available in: http://scielo.sld.cu/pdf/rpr/v20n4/rpr05416.pdf
31. Meza-Prambs A, Vergara-Cabezas R, Encalada-Campos G, Estay-Sepulveda J, Crespo J, Cabezas Caceres C. Ideal treatment of insulin resistance and prediabetes; ^Metformin or exercise? J Sport Heal Res J Sport Heal Res 14 [Internet]. 2019[cited 2024 my 26];(11):139- 54. Available at: http://www.journalshr.com/papers/Vol 11 supplement2/JSHR V11 SUPL2 12.pdf

32. Ceballos-Pomares JC, SoKs-Martmez RA, Quevedo-Carreno A, Lopez Munoz JJD, MORENO-Cortes ML. Insulin resistance and its relationship with biochemical and anthropometric alterations in adolescents with prediabetes. Revista Biomedica [Internet]. 2020 [cited 2024 my 26];31(1). Available from: https://doi.org/10.32776/revbiomed
33. CARRASCo F, GALGANI J, REYES M. La Resistance Syndrome. REV MED CLIN. 2018; 24(5):827-37.
34. Escobar J, Chimal M, Moreno M, Lagunes O, Ortega C, Escobar P. Detection of risk factors for insulin resistance in university students. Acta Med Centro [Internet]. 2018 [cited 2024 my26]; 12(3):332-8. Available at: http://www.revactamedicacentro.sld.cu/index.php/amc/article/view/971/1172
35. Fragozo-Ramos C. Metabolic syndrome: a review of the literature. Med Lab [Internet]. 2022 [cited 2024 my 26];26(1):47-62. Available from: https://medicinaylaboratorio.com/index.php/myl/article/view/559/503
36. Chacon-Valladares P, Valencia-Gutierrez MM. Metabolic syndrome and lifestyles in health personnel in a family medicine unit in Mexico. Cad Aten Primaria [Internet] 2020 [cited 2024 my 26]; 26 (3):4-11. Available at: https://revista.agamfec.com/wp-content/uploads/2021/01/Agamfec 26 3-Orixinal-Shdrome-metab6lico.pdf
37. Vinces-Chong RI, Villamarin-Vaca ON, Tapia-Mieles AM, Gorozabel- Alarcon JM, Delgado-Gorozabel CJ, Vinces-Zambrano MI. Diabetes Mellitus and its serious impact on Uphic complications. Polo del Conoc. 2019; 4(2):181.
38. Casal-Dommguez M, Pinal-Fernandez I. Clinical practice guideline on type 2 diabetes mellitus. Arch Med. 2014; 10(2):1-18.
39. Carrillo-Larco RM, Bernabe-Ortiz A. Type 2 diabetes mellitus in Peru: a systematicreview of prevalence and incidence in the general population. Rev Peru Med Exp Salud Publica. 2019; 36(1):26-36.
40. American Diabetes Association Professional Practice Committee. Standards of medical care in diabetes-2022. Diabetes Care. 2022;45(suppl 1):1-16.7
41. Ministry of Health and Consumer Affairs. Ministry of Health and Social Services. Guia de practica clmica sobre Diabetes Mellitus type 2. Serv Cent Comun del Gob Vasco [Internet]. 2017 [Cited 2024 my 26]; 1 -181. Available in: https://portal.guiasalud.es/wpcontent/uploads/2018/12/GPC 429 Diabetes 2 Osteba compl.pd
42. American Diabetes Association (ADA). Type 2 diabetes guide for clinicians. Redgdps [Internet]. 2022 [cited 2024 my 26]:264. Available from: https://www.redgdps.org/gestor/upload/colecciones/Guia DM2 web.pdf.
43. Meza C, San MartmC , Ruiz J, Frugone C. Pathophysiology of diabeticnephropathy: a literaturereview [Fisiopatolog^a de la nefropaUa diabetica: una revisión de la literatura]. Medwave [Internet]. 2017[cited 2024my26]; 17(1):e6839. Available In: http://dx.doi.org/10.5867/medwave.2017.01.6839
44. Bustillo-Solano EE, Bustillo-Madrigal EE, Perez-Francisco Y, Perez-Sosa R, Brito-Garrta A, Gonzalez-Iglesia A, et al. Prevalence of diabetes mellitus and impaired fasting blood glucose in an area of Sancti Spmitus city. Rev Cubana

Endocrinol [Internet]. 2013 Aug [cited 2024 my29]; 24(2): 107-124. Available in: http://scielo.sld.cu/scielo.php?script=sci arttext&pid=S1561 -29532013000200002&lng=en.

45. Aravinda J. Riskfactors in patientswithtype 2 diabetes in Bengaluru: A retrospectivestudy. World J Diabetes [Internet] 2019[cited 2024 my 26]; 10(4), 241-248.Available from: https://doi.org/10.4239/wjd.v10.i4.241

46. Bohorquez-Moreno C, Barreto-Vasquez M, Muvd-iMuvdi YP, Rodriguez- Sanjuan A, Badillo-Viloria M A, Martmez de la Rosa WA, et al. Modifiable factors and risk of type 2 diabetes mellitus in young adults: a cross-sectional study. Sci. Sick [Internet]. 2020 [cited 2024 my 26]; 26: 14. Available from: https://doi.org/10.29393/ce26-7fmcb70007.

47. Carpio-Troya AC, Camacho-Ullauri ZP, Maldonado-Rengel RE. Diabetes mellitus and diabetic nephropaUa. cietna [Internet]. July 29, 2023 [cited 2024 abr3]; 10(1): 120-137. Disponible in: https://revistas.usat.edu.pe/index.php/cietna/article/view/899

48. Sanchez J, Sanchez N. Epidemiology^a of type 2 diabetes mellitus and its complications. Rev Finlay [Internet]. 2022 Jun [cited 2024 Apr 19]; 12(2):168-176 . in: http://scielo.sld.cu/scielo.php?script=sci arttext&pid=S2221 -24342022000200168&lng=en

49. Castillo HF, Morocho MC, Naranjo GJ. Risk of Diabetes Mellitus type 2 in the health personnel of the Alfredo Noboa Montenegro Hospital. Guaranda- Ecuador. Revista Eugenio Espejo [Internet] 2019 [cited 2024 my 29; 13(2): 42-52. en: https://eugenioespejo.unach.edu.ec/index.php/EE/article/view/148

50. Khan, M. A., Hashim, M. J., King, J. K., Govender, R. D., Mustafa, H., &Kaabi, J. A. (2020). Epidemiolog^a of type 2 diabetes: global burden of disease and projected trends. J EpidemiolGlob Health, 100(1).

51. American Diabetes Association. ADA. Standards of care in diabetes. ADA guideline, 2023. Diabetes Care [Internet] 2023 [cited 2024 my29]; 4 (suppl. 1). Available from: ADA . Available from: https://mariamontanavivas.wordpress.com/2022/12/14/estandares-de- diabetes-care-guide-guide-all-2023-free/

52. Serna LM, Pineda N, Garcia AM, Aguirre M, Alfaro JM, Balthazar V, et al. Nefropatia diabetica. MEDICINA UPB [Internet]. 2009 [cited 2023 Jan 28]; 28(1): 42-53 . en: https://bibliotecadigital.udea.edu.co/dspace/bitstream/10495/26229/1/Higuit aLina 2009 NefropatiasdiabeticasDiabetesMellitus.pdf

53. Sanchez B, Vega V, Gomez N, Vilema G. Case-control study on risk factors for type 2 diabetes mellitus in older adults. Revista Universidad y Sociedad [Internet]. 2020 [cited 2024 my 29]; 12(4): 156-164. Available en: http://scielo.sld.cu/scielo.php?script=sci arttext&pid=S2218-36202020000400156&lng=es&tlng=es

54. Leiva A, Martmez M, Petermann F, Garrido A, Poblete F, D^az X, et al. Factors associated with the development of type 2 diabetes mellitus in Chile. Nutr Hosp

[Internet]. 2018 Apr [cited 2024 my 29]; 35(2): 400-407. Available from: http://scielo.isciii.es/scielo.php?script=sci arttext&pid=S0212-16112018000200400&lng=es. https://dx.doi.org/10.20960/nh.1434 .
55. Cipriani E, Quintanilla A. Type 2 diabetes mellitus and insulin resistance. Rev Med Hered [Internet]. 2010 [cited 2024 my 29]; 21(3): 160-71. Available in: http://www.scielo.org.pe/scielo.php?script=sciarttext&pid=S1018-130X2010000300008
56. Albaro F, Martmez A, Gorriz L. Significance of early determination of microalbuminuria in global vascular risk and diabetic nephropathy. Nefrologia [Internet] 2005 [cited 2024 my 29]; 25 suppl.4). Available from: file:///C:/Users/HP/Downloads/X0211699505031341 .pdf.
57. Gonzalez-Fajardo I, Borrego-Carmona C, Morera-Rojas BP, D^az-Padilla D. Prevalence of microalbuminuria in obese and hypertensive children and its relationship with cardiovascular risk factors. Rev Medical Sciences [Internet]. 2015 Aug [cited 2023 my 29]; 19(4): 604-618. Available from: http://scielo.sld.cu/scielo.php?script=sci arttext&pid=S1561 -
58. Ortega-Filartiga EA, Prevalence and clinical characteristics of diabetic nephropathy. Rev Nac (Itaugua) [Internet]. 2013 [cited 2024 my 29];5(1):18- 27. Available en: http://scielo.iics.una.py/scielo.php?script=sci arttext&pid=S2072- 817420130001000
59. Viberti GC, Jarrett RJ, Mahmud U, Hill RD, Argyropoulos A, Keen H. Microalbuminuria as a predictor of clinical nephropathy in insulin-dependent diabetes mellitus. Lancet [Internet]. 1982 [cited 2024 my 29]; 319(8287):1430-2. Disponible en: https://www.sciencedirect.com/science/article/pii/S0140673682924503
60. Vergara-Arana A, Martmez-Castelao A, Gorriz-Teruel JL, Alvaro-Moreno F de, Navarro-Gonzalez JF, Soler-Romeo MJ. Diabetic Renal Disease: Albuminuria and Progression. Nefrolog^a al D^a [Internet]. 2020 [cited 2024 my 29]: [ca. 8p.]. Available from: https://www.nefrologiaaldia.org/esarticulo- enfermedad-diabetica-renal-albuminuria-progresion-292
61. Jimenez A, Aguilar C, Rojas R, Hernandez M. Diabetes mellitus type 2 and frequency of actions for its prevention and control. Salud Publ Mex[Internet]. 2013 [cited 2024 my 29]; 55: S137-43. Available from: https://www.scielo.org.mx/scielo.php?script=sci arttext&pid=S0036-36342013000800010
62. Prada S, Marrugo M, Arcia L, Vega G, Ricardo L, Ballesteros E, et al. Diabetic kidney disease: state of the art. Archives of Medicine. 2022; 18(6):1. Available in: https://dialnet.unirioja.es/servlet/articulo?codigo=8540250
63. Villena A. Risk factors for diabetic nephropathy. Acta Med Peru [Internet]. 2021 [Accessed 2024 my 29]; 38(4). Available in: http://dx.doi.org/10.35663/amp.2021.384.2256.
64. Perez CR and Mallma YM. Lifestyle in older adults with type II diabetes mellitus in a housing complex in Lima. Agora [Internet]. 2021 [cited2024 my 29]; 8(2): 20-6. Available from: https://www.revistaagora.com/index.php/cieUMA/article/ view/189

65. Vazquez A, Cervantes T, SoKs E, Franco G, Valencia E, Centeno S, et al. Self-care strategies in patients with type 2 diabetes mellitus. Rev Esp Med Quir [Internet]. 2012 [cited 2024 my 29]; 17(2): 94 -9. Available from:
https://www.medigraphic.com/cgi-bin/new/summary.cgi?IDARTICLE=35156
66. Serra M. Actualization on antidiabetic drugs and risk cardiovascular. Rev Urug Cardiol [Internet]. 2016 Dec [cited 2024 my 19]; 31(3): 522-546. Disponible en: http://www.scielo.edu.uy/scielo.php?script=sci arttext&pid=S1688-04202016000300014&lng=es
67. Criteria for the use of non-insulin antidiabetics in patients with Type 2 Diabetes Mellitus. Madrid: Comunidad de Madrid, Servicio Madrileno de Salud, Consejeria de Sanidad; Feb 2020 [cited 2024 my 29]. 86p . Criteria: n10). Available en:
http://www.madrid.org/bvirtual/BVCM050241 .pdf
68. Cruz R, Fuentes O, Gutierrez O, Garay R, Aguila O. Diabetic nephropathy in type 2 diabetic patients. Rev Cubana Med. 2011; 50(1): 29-39.
69. Villena Pacheco Arturo. Risk factors for diabetic nephropathy. Acta med. Peru [Internet]. 2021 Oct [cited 2024 Jun 05] ; 38(4): 283-294. Available in: http:/www.scielo.org.pe/scielo.php?script=sci_arttext&pid=S1728-59172021000400283&lng=es. Epub04-Feb-2022 .
http://dx.doi.org/10.35663/amp.2021.384.2256
70. Yamazaki T, Mimura I, Tanaka T, Nangaku M. Treatment of Diabetic Kidney disease: current and future. Diabetes Metab J [internet] 2021 [cited 2024 my 29]; 45(1): 11-26. Available from: https://pubmed.ncbi.nlm.nih.gov/33508907/
71. GBD Chronic Kidney Disease Collaboration. Global, regional, and nationalburden of chronickidneydisease, 1990-2017; a systematic analysis forthe global burden of diseasestudy 2017. Lancet [Internet] 2020 [cited 2024my29]; 395: 709-33 . in:
https://www.thelancet.com/journals/lancet/issue/vol395no10225/PIIS0140-6736(20)X0009-2
72. Calle A, Criollo L, Salinas S, Tello J, Altamirano C, Bermeo M. Risk factors for diabetic nephropathy in adults: update of the literature. Archivos Venezolanos de Farmacolog^a y Terapeutica [Internet] 2022 [cited 2024 my 29]; 41(3): 172-184. Available from: https://www.revistaavft.com/images/revistas/2022/avft_3_2022/4_risk factors nephropatia.pdf.
73. Toala Y, Leon M, Pin A. Prevalence of type 2 diabetes mellitus and its risk factors in Latin American adults. MQR Research [Internet] 2023 [cited 2024 my 29]; 7(1), 742-763. Available from:
https:ZZdoi.org/10.56048/MQR20225.7.1.2023.742-763
74. Fuentes-de-la-Rosa Y, D^az-Cabrera J, D^az-Calzada M, Rodriguez-Sardinas L, Perez-Alvarez Y. Characterization of the metabolic syndrome in type 2 diabetics treated at the Provincial Center of Pinar del Rfo. Rev Ciencias Medicas de Pinar del Rfo [Internet]. 2023 [cited 2024 my 29]; 27: [approx. 5p .]. Available en:
https://revcmpinar.sld.cu/index.php/publicaciones/article/view/5861

75. Sanchez-Alvarez GA, Betancourt-Reyes GL, Betancourt-Betancourt G de J. Clinical-epidemiological characterization of patients with type 2 diabetes mellitus and microalbuminuria. Rev Med Electron [Internet] 2023[cited 2024 my29]. in: https://revmedicaelectronica.sld.cu/index.php/rme/article/view/5045
76. Russo-Maria P, Grande-Ratti MF, Burgos MA, Molaro AA, Bonella MB. Prevalence of diabetes, epidemiological characteristics and vascular complications. Arch Cardiol Mex [Internet]. 2023 March [cited 2024 my 12]; 93(1): 30-36 . in: http://www.scielo.org.mx/scielo.php?script=sciarttext&pid=S1405-99402023000100030&lng=es. Epub24-Feb-2023 . https://doi.org/10.24875/acm.21000410.
77. International Diabetes Federation. IDF Diabetes Atlas. 9ed. 2019 [Internet]. International Diabetes Federation;2019 [cited 2024 my 29]. Available in: https://www.diabetesatlas.org/upload/resources/material/20200302 133352 2406-IDF-ATLAS-SPAN-BOOK.pdf
78. Avila-Gonzalez Z, Lopez-Pena Y. Addressing diabetes mellitus: prevention strategies from current scientific evidence. LATAM [Internet]. November 24, 2023 [cited 2024 my 12];4(5):1189-1202. Available from: http://latam.redilat.org/index.php/lt/article/view/1387
79. Penafiel-Cruz GK, Villa-Mej^a JA, Barcia-Menendez R. Prevalence and morbidity of diabetes mellitus type 2 diabetes mellitus in older adults in Latin America. MQRIresearch [Internet]. 2023 on 18 [cited 2024 my 12];7(1):248-6. Available from: MQRInvestigar [Internet]. in: https://www.investigarmqr.com/ojs/index.php/mqr/article/view/165
80. Tellez-Ramos CM, Florian DA, Reyes-Garay N. Factors associated with chronic kidney disease at Carlos Roberto Huembes Hospital. Rev Torreon Universitario [Internet]. 2023 [cited 2024 my 12];12(35):93-100. Available in: https://revistasnicaragua.cnu.edu.ni/index.php/torreon/article/view/8269
81. Hernandez-Zambrano SM, Carrillo-Algarra AJ, Linares-Rodriguez LV, Martmez-Ruiz AL, Nunez-Yaguna MF. Sociodemographic and clinical characterization of patients with chronic kidney disease in condition of pluripathology and their caregivers. Enferm Nefrol [Internet]. 2021 [cited 2023 Oct. 24];24(1):[approx. 12 screens]. Available in: https://scielo.isciii.es/pdf/enefro/v24n1/2255-3517- enefro-24-01-06.pdf
82. Mederos-Borroto Y, Tiza-Perez Y, Perez-Valencia B. Educational intervention to modify levels of knowledge about chronic kidney disease in diabetic patients. Medicent Electron [Internet] 2024 [cited 2024 my 29]; 28: e4129. Available from: Medicent Electron [Internet] 2024 [cited 2024 my 29]; 28: e4129. in: https://medicentro.sld.cu/index.php/medicentro/article/view/4129/3335
83. Mohammedi K, Chalmers J, Herrington W, Li Q, Mancia G, Marre M, et al. Associations between bodymassindex andtherisk of renal events in patients with type 2 diabetes. Nutr Diabetes [Internet] 2018 [Cited 2024 my 29]; 8:7. Available from: DOI 10.1038/s41387-017-0012.
84. Jitraknatee J, Ruengorn C, Nochaiwong S. Prevalence and risk factors of chronic kidney diseaseamong type 2diabetes patients: a cross-sectional study. sectionalstudy in primarycarepractice. Sci Rep. 2020 Apr 10; 10(1):6205. doi: 10.1038/s41598-020-63443-4. PMID :32277150; PMCID:

PMC7148316.
85. Polanco N, Rodriguez F. Results of an early detection program for diabetic nephroparia. Med Interna Mex [Internet]. 2019 [cited 2024my29]; 35(2): 198-207. Available en: http://www.scielo.org.mx/scielo.php?script=sciarttext&pid=S0186-48662019000200198
86. Gheith O, Farouk N, Nampoory N, Halim MA, Al-Otaibi T. Diabetic kidney disease: world wide difference of prevalence and riskf actors. J Nephropharmacol [Internet] 2016 [cited 2024my29]; 5(1): p. 49-56. Available in: https://www.ncbi.nlm.nih.gov/pmc/articles/PMC5297507/pdf/npj-5-49.pdf
87. Radcliffe NJ, Seah J, Clarke M, Maclsaac RJ, Jerums G & Ekinci El. Clinical predictive factors in diabetic kidney disease progression. J Diabetes Investig [Internet] 2017 [cited 2024 my 29]; 8: p. 6-18. Available from: https://pubmed.ncbi.nlm.nih.gov/27181363/
88. Zuo PY, Chen XL, Liu YW, Zhang R, He XX, Liu CY. Non-HDL- HDL-cholesterolto HDL-cholesterol ratio as anindependentrisk factor forthedevelopment of chronickidneydisease. Nutr Metab Cardiovasc Dis[Internet] 2015 [Cited 2024 my 29]; 25 (6): 582-7. Available from: https:ZZdoi.org/10.1016/j.numecd.2015.03.003.
89. Aleman G, Gomez I, Reques L, Rosado J, Polentinos E, Rodriguez R. Prevalence and risk of progression of chronic kidney disease in diabetic and hypertensive patients followed in primary care in the Community of Madrid. Nefrolog^a [Internet] 2017[cited 2024 my 29] ; 37 (3): 338-54. Available from: https://scielo.isciii.es/pdf/nefrologia/v37n3/0211 - 6995-nefrologia-37-03-00343.pdf.
90. Lopez-Simarro F. Prevention of chronic kidney disease in people with diabetes mellitus. Diabetes Practica [Internet] 2023 [: 1(Suppl Extr 2):1- 50. https://doi.Org/10.52102/diabetpract.renal.art6
91. Tziomalos K, Athyros VG. Diabetic nephropathy: new risk factors and improvements in diagnosis. Rev Diabetic Studies [Internet] 2015 [cited 2024my29]; 12(1-2). 67. Available In: https://pubmed.ncbi.nlm.nih.gov/26676664/
92. Kajiwara A, Kita A, Saruwatari J, Hiroko M, Kawata Y, Morita K, et al. Sex differences in the renal function decline of patientswithtype 2 diabetes. J Diabetes Res [Internet] 2016 [Cited 2024 my 29]:4626382. Available from: https:ZZdoi.org/10.1155/2016/4626382.
93. Wagner F, Eshetie S, Kibret GD, Zegeye A, Dessie G, Mulugeta H, et al. Diabetic nephropathy and hypertension in diabetes patients of sub-Saharancountries: a systematicreview and meta-analysis. BMC Res Notes [Internet]2018[cited 2024 my 29];11:565. Available from: https://doi.org/10.1186/s13104-018-3670-5
94. Garofalo C, Borrelli S, Minutolo R, Chiodini P, De Nicola L, Conte G. A systematicreviewandmeta-analysissuggestsobesitypredictsonsetofchronickidneydisease in the general population. Kidney Int.[Internet] 2017[cited 2024 my 29] ; 91 (5): 1224-35. Available from: https://doi: 10.1016/j.kint.2016.12.013. Epub 2017 Feb 7. PMID: 28187985.

95. DurrerSchutz D, Busetto L, Dicker D. EuropeanPracticalandPatient-CentredGuidelinesforAdultObesity Management in PrimaryCare. ObesFacts. 2019; 12 (1): 40-66. Disponible in: https://doi.org/10.1159/000496183
96. Xia J, Wang L, Ma Z, Zhong L, Wang Y, Gao Y, et al. Cigarette smoking and chronickidneydisease in the general population: a systematicreview and meta-analysis of prospectivecohortstudies. Nephrol Dial Transplant. [Internet] 2017 Mar 1 [cited 2024 my 29];32(3):475-487. Available from: https://doi: 10.1093/ndt/gfw452.
97. Yuan HC, Yu QT, Bai H, Xu HZ, Gu P, Chen LY. Alcohol intake and risk of chronickidneydisease: resultsfrom a systematicreview and doseresponse meta-analysis. Eur J ClinNutr [Internet] 2021 Nov [cited 2024 my 29]; 75(11):1555-1567. Available from: https://doi: 10.1038/s41430-021- 00873-x
98. Kruzel-Davila E, Wasser WG, Aviram S, Skorecki K. APOL1 nephropathy: frome gene tomechanisms of kidneyinjury. Nephrol Dial Transplant.[Internet] 2016 [cited 2023 my 29]; 31: p. 349. Available from: https://doi: 10.1093/ndt/gfu391. Epub 2015 Jan 5. PMID: 25561578.
99. Liao LN, Li TCh, Li Ch, LiuChS, Lin WY, LinChH, et al. Geneticrisk score forriskprediction of diabeticnephropathy in Han Chinesetype 2 diabetes patients. Scientific Reports [Internet] 2019 [cited 2024 my 29]; 9:19897. Available from: https://doi: 10.1038/s41598-019-56400-3. PMID: 31882689; PMCID: PMC6934611.
100. HungChCH, Lin HYS, Hwang DY, KuolCh, Chiu YW, Lim LM, et al. Diabetic retinopathy and clinical parameters favoring the presence of diabetic nephropathy could predict renal outcome in patients with diabetic kidney disease. Sci Rep. 2017 Apr 21;7(1):1236. Available at: https://doi: 10.1038/s41598-017-01204-6. PMID: 28432319; PMCID: PMC5430840
101. Liang S, Zhang XG, Cai GY, Zhu HY, Zhou JH, Wu J, et al. Identifying parametersto distinguish non-diabetic renal diseases from diabetic nephropathy in patients withtype 2 diabetes mellitus: a meta-analysis. PLoS ONE [Internet] 2013 [cited 2024 my 29]; 8(5): e64184. Available from: https://doi: 10.1371/journal. pone.0064184.
102. Landrove-Rodriguez O, Morejon-Giraldoni A, Venero-Fernandez S, Suarez-Medina R, Almaguer-Lopez M, Pallarols-Marino E, et al. Non communicable diseases: risk factors and actions fortheir prevention and control in Cuba. Rev Panam Salud Publica [Internet] 2018 Apr [cited 2024 my 29] 24; 42:e23. Available from: https://doi: 10.26633/RPSP.2018.23. PMID: 31093052; PMCID: PMC6386105.
103. Herrera Valdes R, Almaguer Lopez M, Chipi Cabrera JA, Perez-Oliva D^az JF, Landrove Rodriguez O, Marmol Sonora A. Prevalence and incidence of chronic kidney disease in Cuba. Clin Nephrol. 2020 Supplement-Jan; 93(1):68-71. https://doi:10.5414/CNP92S111.PMID: 31549629.
104. Mazzucco G, Bertani T, Fortunato M et al. Differentpatterns of renal damage in type 2 diabetes mellitus: a multicentricstudyon 393 biopsies. Am J Kidney Dis. 2002Apr ;39(4):713-20 Available in : https://doi.org/10.1053/ajkd.2002.31988
105. Garces S, Dayly Y. Nursing educational intervention to improve the knowledge of adherence to treatment in patients with chronic kidney disease at the Daniel

Alcides Carrion Hospital [graduate thesis]. [Lima, Peru]: Universidad Cesar Vallejo; 2019. [cited 2024 my 29]. Available from: https://repositorio.ucv.edu.pe/handle/20.500.12692/39945

106. Burgos-Jimenez E, Melendez-Balderrama MA, Meza-Coronado E, Agramon-Cota KG, Pereyra-Hernandez MC, Martmez-MenchacaNL . Impact of an intervention aimed at increasing knowledge of kidney disease on the timely initiation of renal replacement therapy. Rev Soc Esp Enferm Nefrol [Internet]. 2011 [cited 2024 my 24];4(4):[approx. 6 screens]. at: https://scielo.isciii.es/pdf/nefro/v14n4/05 original4.pdf

107. Robalino-Rivadeneira ME, Urdaneta-Carruyo GM, Chilquina-Cabay RJ, Paca-Pilco EA, Chimbo-Bayas WG, Rea-Manobanda MA. Level of knowledge about chronic kidney disease in patients, relatives and nursing staff. Rev Cubana Reumatol [Internet]. 2021 [cited 2024 my 24];23(3):[approx. 14 screens]. Available from: http://scielo.sld.cu/pdf/rcur/v23n3/1817-5996-rcur-23-03- e233.pdf

108. Valverde-Chocho LE, Zari-Alvarez MA. Knowledge, attitudes and practices on self-care of patients undergoing renal replacement therapy at the DialiLife centre, Cuenca 2016 [thesis]. [Cuenca- Ecuador]: Universidad de Cuenca; 2016[cited 2024 my 29]. Available from: http://dspace.ucuenca.edu.ec/handle/123456789/25647

109. Gongora-Gomez O, Riveron-Carralero W, Saavedra-Munoz L, Bauta-Milord R, Gomez-Vazquez Y. Educational intervention on chronic renal failure in patients with type 2 diabetes mellitus. Univ Med Pinarena [Internet]. 2019 [cited 2024 my 29]; 15(2):[approx. 9 p.]. Available from: https://revgaleno.sld.cu/index.php/ump/article/view/339/pdf

110. Huaman-Carhuas L, Gutierrez-Crespo HF. Impact of nursing intervention on self-care in patients with advanced chronic kidney disease. Enferm Nefrol [Internet]. 2021 mzo[cited 2024 my 29]];24(1):[approx. 9p .]. Available in: http://scielo.isciii.es/scielo.php?script=sci arttext&pid=S2254-28842021000100007&lng=es

111. Vera-Brand J, Aroca-Martmez G, Fonseca-Angulo R, Rodriguez-Vera D. Level of knowledge of patients with CKD about their disease in Barranquilla Colombia. Rev Latinoam Hipertens [Internet]. 2019 [cited 2024 my 29]; 14(2):[approx. 7 p.]. Available from: https://www.redalyc.org/journal/1702/170263775002/html/

112. Lopez-Cata FJ, Matos-Santisteban M, Inclan-Rodriguez D, Escobar-Paz 1, Valdes-Miranda V. Intervencion educativa en adultos mayores sobre la enfermedad renal cronica. Univ Med Pinarena [Internet]. 2020 [cited 2024 my29]; 17(1):[approx. 10p .]. Available from: Univ Med Pinarena [Internet] . in: https://revgaleno.sld.cu/index.php/ump/article/view/488/pd

113. Duzalan OB, Pakyuz SC. Educational interventions forim proveddiet and fluid management in haemodialysis patients. An interventional study. J Pak Med Assoc[Internet] 2018 Apr[cited 2024 my 29];68(4):532-537. Available from: https://pubmed.ncbi.nlm.nih.gov/29808040/PMID: 29808040.

114. Dos Santos KK, Lucas TC, Gloria JCR, do Carmo-Pereira A, Junior GDCR, Lara MO. Epidemiological profile of chronic renal patients in treatment. Journal of

Nursing UFPE / Revista de Enfermagem UFPE.
[Internet] 2018 [cited 2024 my 29]; 12(9). Available from:
https://doi.Org/10.5205/1981 -8963-v12i9a234508p2293-2300-2018
115. Sanchez-Gonzalez JC, Martmez-Marthez C, Bethencourt-Fernandez D, Pablos-Lopez M. Valoracion de los conocimientos que tienen los pacientes en hemodialisisis acerca de su tratamiento. Enferm Nefrol [Internet]. 2015March [cited 2024 my 29]; 18(1): 23-30. Available from:
http://scielo.isciii.es/scielo.php?script=sci arttext&pid=S2254-28842015000100004&lng=es https://dx.doi.org/10.4321/S2254-28842015000100004.

Annexes

Annex 1. Informed Consent

I: hereby certify that

I was informed about:

That this is an investigation to improve the information level of type 2 diabetic patients to prevent chronic kidney disease. That my participation will be safe for me. That the research is beneficial to me and will help me to achieve the vision of the future for the prevention of chronic kidney disease.

That I can withdraw whenever I wish without any kind of reprisal against me.

That I have to answer questions about personal issues and planned activities, and I am assured that it will be completely confidential.

In accordance with the above, I confirm my willingness to participate in the research:

Participant Researcher

Annex 2. Data form for the review of individual medical histories and family files.

1. Age. .
2. Gender. Female Male
3. Schooling.
   Primary
   Secondary
   Pre-university

Medium technician
   University

4. Body mass index:
   Underweight. Less than 18.5.
   Normal weight: (from 18.5-24.9)
   Overweight (25.0-29.9)
   Obesity (greater than or equal to 30)
5. Time of evolution of DM since diagnosis.

5 years old or less.

From 6 to 10 years

Older than 10 years.

6. Risk factors for CKD.
   Arterial hypertension
   Dyslipidaemia

Ischaemic CardiopaUa
   Obesity

Smoking
   Consumption of alcoholic beverages
   Consumption of nephrotoxic drugs
   Family history of kidney disease
   Other

Annex 3: Gua de observation of albuminuria as an early marker of renal damage.

Objective: To identify whether albuminuria exists in patients with type 2 DM participating in the study.

Means of observation: gua de observation.
Conditions of observation direct observation of the results by the researcher.
Mark a cross (X) in the Negative or Positive boxes corresponding to the presence or absence of microalbuminuria in type 2 diabetic patients.

Renal damage marker	Results	
	Negative (less than 20 mg/l)	Positive (between 20-200 mg/)l
Albuminuria		

Annex 4. Diagnostic and evaluative questionnaire.

1. Age.
2. Sex: F M
3. Do you consider that diabetes mellitus (DM) can be a cause of chronic kidney disease (CKD)?
   Yes No
4. Listed below are several risk factors ^Which ones do you think may cause CKD? Mark with an (x) the ones you think are correct.

a Arterial hypertension
b Dyslipidaemia
c Eating very spicy foods. spicy foods.
d Obesity
e Practice of physical exercises exercises
f Smoking
g Consumption of alcoholic alcoholic beverages
h Drink plenty of water.
i Family history of kidney disease
j Others ^Which ones?

5. Considering the main clinical manifestations of CKD, state 4 symptoms that you are aware of.
6. What complications can patients suffering from CKD have? Mark with an (x) what you think is correct.

a Arterial hypertension
b Acute gastritis
c Malnutrition
d Anemia
e Arthritis
f Death
g Metabolic acidosis
h Pneumoma
i Cardiovascular disease
j Others ^Which ones?

7. Do you think your actions could prevent CKD?
   Yes No
8. Name 4 steps you could take to prevent CKD

<u>Annex 5.</u> Instructions for assessing the questionnaire in Annex 4

The questionnaire will consist of 8 questions, of which questions 1 and 2 will not receive marks as these questions do not measure knowledge of the subject in the sample to be studied. Questions 3 and 7 are worth 10 points and the rest of the questions are worth 20 points for a total of 100 points and will be evaluated as follows: Question 3: Coast of two possible answers. If you answer **Yes**, you get 10 points. If you answer **No,** you get no points.

Question 4: There are 10 items, each worth 2 marks. Correct items: a, b, d, e, f, g, h, i. In the case of item j, the correctness of the answer is assessed.

Question 5: Each answer will be worth 5 marks.

Question 6: There are 10 items, each worth 2 marks. Correct items: a, c, d, f, g, i. In the case of item j, the correctness of the answer is assessed.

Question 7: Coast of two possible answers. If you answer **Yes**, you get 10 points. If you answer **No,** you get no points.

Question 8: 4 measures are requested. Each of them will be worth 5 marks.

<u>Annex 6.</u> Focus group guide:

A thesis is being carried out on an educational programme to prevent CKD in type 2 diabetic patients in the 47th and 48th family doctor's offices of the XX Aniversario polyclinic, Santa Clara municipality, Villa Clara province. It will be of great value to know your criteria in relation to the topics presented in continuation. Your collaboration is needed to acquire information on the following aspects related to the subject:

> Identification of the needs related to the level of information to prevent CKD in type 2 diabetic patients.

> Health promotion on E.

> Impact of the level of information about CKD on CKD prevention in type 2 diabetic patients.

Location:

Time:

Maximum duration 60 minutes.

<u>Central Theme</u>: The level of information to prevent chronic kidney disease (CKD) in type 2 diabetic patients.

<u>Objective</u>: To collect criteria from various specialists in the focus group regarding the topics of interest for the research, in order to create a product that is comprehensible, with appropriate content on the level of information to prevent CKD in type 2 diabetic patients.

<u>Questions:</u>

> In order for the type 2 diabetic patients under study to have a solid basis of information on how to prevent CKD, what aspects do you think should not be missing for the prevention of this disease?

> What could be the reasons that type 2 diabetic patients have little information about CKD and do not know how to apply this information for the prevention of CKD?

> What would you suggest to improve the level of information about CKD in type 2 diabetic patients?

> What do you consider to be the main issues that type 2 diabetic patients should know about CKD?

> How do you think it is most feasible to provide them with this information?
> Mention the main contents that you consider should be taught in an educational programme, considering the target group of patients.

Annex 7. Guide for the Nominal Group:

Theme: Related to the design of the educational programme to prevent chronic kidney disease (CKD) in type 2 diabetic patients in the 47th and 48th family medical offices of the XX Aniversario polyclinic, Santa Clara municipality, Villa Clara province.

Objective: To develop the design of an educational programme related to timely actions on the level of information to prevent chronic kidney disease (CKD) in type 2 diabetic patients in the 47th and 48th family medical offices of the XX Aniversario polyclinic, Santa Clara municipality, Villa Clara province.

Location:

Time:

With a maximum duration of 60 minutes.

The topic to be discussed is raised. Start with open questions.

Mention the main difficulties you consider to exist with regard to this issue in the sample under study. Express your views on this issue.

Questions:

> What actions would be necessary to modify the needs identified?
> ^What would be the themes of the activities?
> ^Knows how to increase the level of information to prevent chronic kidney disease (CKD) in type 2 diabetic patients.
> What techniques do you propose for delivering the proposed actions?
> Could an educational programme help to solve the problems encountered?
> Are there conditions for the design and subsequent implementation of an educational programme in this sample?
> What characteristics should the educational programme for this group have according to their needs?
> Tick as many options as you think we could contribute to improving information on the subject in the type 2 diabetic patients under study?

In the office.

On the ground (home)

Through educational activities planned and coordinated with the Basic Health Team, providing updated information on the subject with images and explanations for patients to access it.

> Please indicate the option through which you think it would be most effective for the information to be provided to the type 2 diabetic patients included in the study. Mark up to 4.

Videos.	Dramatised.
Talks.	Games.
Educational software.	Documents.
Radio.	Conversation.
TV.	Posters and leaflets

Annex 8. Specialists' criteria on the designed educational programme.

In order to evaluate the designed educational programme, the method of evaluation by criteria of specialists, who qualify as such, is applied by means of a process of intentional sampling of key informants with recognised experience as experts in the subject and scientific prestige.

An information process is carried out to form the sample as follows:

> A first degree specialist in Nephrology with more than 10 years of professional experience, lecturer and assistant professor.

> A first degree specialist in Endocrinology with more than 10 years of professional experience, lecturer and assistant professor.

> A first degree specialist in Internal Medicine with more than 10 years of professional experience, lecturer and assistant professor.

> A first degree specialist in General Comprehensive Medicine, with more than 10 years of professional and teaching experience and assistant professors.

> A second degree specialist in General Comprehensive Medicine with more than 30 years of professional and teaching experience.

> A graduate in psychology with the teaching category of instructor.

> A Bachelor of Education with teaching experience, with 25 years of teaching experience

They are considered as evaluative categories:

> Accepted: When 86% to 100% of the consulted specialists evaluated the requested aspects with 4 or 5 and no aspect was evaluated by the specialists with less than 3.

> Accepted with recommendations: When between 70% and 85% of the consulted specialists evaluated the requested aspects out of 4 or 5 and no aspect was evaluated with less than 3.

> Not Accepted: When the results do not conform to the above definition.

In order to carry out the assessment, the specialists will have to fill in the table on the basis of the indications provided and after delivery of the designed product.

It is explained to them that the evaluative categories are to be given in ascending order and it is specified that if it is less than 5 it is expressed below the table which aspect leads them to make decisions.

Operational definitions given in the evaluation for each aspect:

Structure: Whether it is in line with actions to increase the level of knowledge to prevent chronic kidney disease (CKD) in type 2 diabetic patients.

Relevance: Whether the way in which the actions are conceived respond to the difficulties identified in the diagnosis.

Utility: If the product that was designed responds to an identified and unresolved problem.

Feasibility: Whether the actions can be implemented in practice.

Scientific value: If the results obtained are the result of scientific research, carried out through a rigorous research process.

No	Aspects to Evaluate	1	2	3	4	5
1	Structure					
2	Relevance					
3	Utility					

4	Feasibility					
5	Scientific value					

Note: The rating ranges are 5(excellent), 4(good), 3(fair), 2(fair).
1(Bad)
Teaching Category
Academic Level
1. ^How do you consider the actions of the educational intervention programme?
Adequate Not adequate.
The following aspects are taken into account:

> Proposed objectives
> Selection of the aspects it addresses
> Forms of information organisation.
> Suggested techniques and procedures

2-6 What positive and negative aspects do you see in this programme?
3-Suggestions and recommendations to enrich and improve this methodology.

GENERAL DATA OF THE RESPONDENT

Name and surname
Workplace
Positions held
Years of experience in working life
Years of experience as a specialist
Years of research experience
Scientific degree achieved
Have you conducted research on this topic? Y^ No
Criteria to be taken into account when selecting the sample:
> Teachers with main teaching categories.
> Be linked to the specialities of General Comprehensive Medicine, Endocrinology, Nephrology, Internal Medicine and Psychology.
> Master's degree and/or doctorate in science.

ANNEX 9: EDUCATIONAL PROGRAMME

Title: Protecting my health

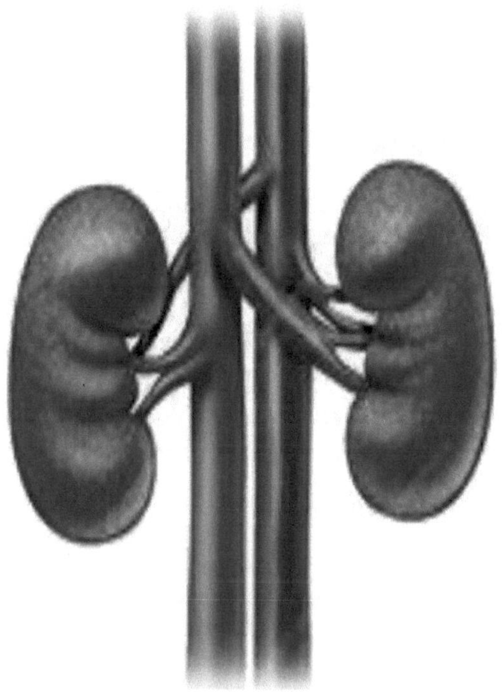

Title: Protecting my health

INTRODUCTION

Diabetes mellitus (DM) type 2 is a chronic disease that represents a public health problem in both first world and underdeveloped countries; it generates a high social and economic impact that leads to a decrease in the quality of life of those who suffer from it, as well as to the loss of years of productive life and potential life span as a consequence of its complications. [1]

Diabetic kidney disease (DKD) is a microvascular complication that affects approximately 35% of patients with type 2 diabetes mellitus, frequently progresses to chronic kidney disease (CKD) with the need for dialysis or kidney transplantation and is one of the most important causes of mortality in patients with type 2 DM. [2]

Early recognition of risk factors for the progression of CKD can be decisive in reducing morbidity and mortality. Some of them are not modifiable: family history, genetics, gender, age at diagnosis and duration of DM. Others are: control of blood glucose and blood pressure, maintaining a healthy lipid profile, avoiding or quitting smoking, reducing alcohol consumption, physical activity and following a balanced diet. As a CKD prevention measure, the American Diabetes Association (ADA) recommends at least annual albuminuria screening. [3]

It is essential to bear in mind that beliefs about health and disease, as well as the patient's perspective on them, influence compliance or non-compliance with behavioural and self-care recommendations. It has been shown that by educating the patient, adequate control of DM is achieved, allowing them to have a practically normal life, both in terms of quality and duration.[2,3]

RATIONALE

In response to this health problem, Cuba has a National Diabetes Programme with the following objectives:

J Decrease the effects of DM on the population.

J Decrease morbidity due to DM.

J Decrease premature mortality from DM.

J Reduce the frequency and severity of acute and chronic complications of MD.

J Improve the quality of life of people with MD.

CKD is a terrible complication in patients with DM. Detecting and treating it contributes to improving the health of the general population.[4]

In view of the above, there is an urgent need to take an active role in informing the public about the magnitude of the problem of diabetes and kidney disease, to encourage early detection and evaluation of these patients, and to try to prevent what is essentially a preventable disease. In recent years, science has shown beyond doubt that the progression of kidney disease can be prevented or slowed. Likewise, it is possible to prevent the onset of DM, as well as to slow and even halt the progression of DKD, with proper control of blood glucose and blood pressure. Early detection of albuminuria in these patients would allow intervention at early stages of DKD and thus prevent or slow the progression to CKD.

The design of the educational programme aims to provide clear and scientific messages so that the approaches have the expected effect. In addition, it is intended to facilitate some participatory techniques according to the different themes of work to achieve individual modes of action that promote the control of those factors that can be modified to achieve a healthy life.

OBJECTIVES

<u>General objective</u>

Raise the level of information for patients with type 2 DM to prevent CKD).

<u>Specific objectives</u>

1. To know the general facts about DM and CKD.
2. Determine the risk factors that may cause CKD in children and adolescents.

diabetic patients.

3. To outline the main clinical manifestations and complications.

that are presented in the ERC.

4. Explain measures to prevent CKD.

SCOPE: Patients with type 2 DM.

TARGET POPULATION: Patients with type 2 DM.

ORGANISATION OF THE PROGRAMME

The programme is carried out in two stages, an intensive stage and a reinforcement stage. It is aimed at 60 patients with type 2 DM from the 47th and 48th family doctor's offices of the XX Aniversario polyclinic, selected to participate in the research, and is carried out in the 28 de Enero primary school. Taking into account the main difficulties diagnosed, the aim is to broaden and strengthen the level of information for diabetic patients in order to prevent CKD.

The intensive stage has a duration of three months, from June to August 2023, five activities are developed with a fortnightly frequency of one hour each, developed as a space for group reflection.

The reinforcement stage is carried out during three consecutive months, from September to November 2023, with a duration of one hour, with the participation of the type 2 diabetic patients included in the study, and is carried out in the 28 de Enero primary school. In the last session, the evaluation is carried out (November 2023) by applying the evaluation questionnaire (Annex 4).

I. DISTRIBUTION OF TOPICS

Intensive stage			
Topics	**First session**	**Second session**	**Total**
Session 1 "Getting to know my illness". Topic 1: Introduction to the educational programme "Protecting my health". General information on DM.	30 minutes	30 minutes	1 hour
Session 2 "How can I get sick? "Theme 2: CKD. General. Risk factors that can cause CKD in patients with type 2 DM.	30 minutes	30 minutes	1 hour
Session 3 "What can I feel? "Topic 3: Main clinical manifestations occurring in CKD.	30 minutes	30 minutes	1 hour
Session 4 "Recognising the danger".	30 minutes	30 minutes	1 hour
Theme 4: Complications that occur in CKD.			
Session 5 "I am preparing to improve my health" Theme 5: Measures to prevent CKD.	30 minutes	30 minutes	1 hour
Reinforcement stage			
First month: General information on DM and CKD. Risk factors that may cause CKD in patients with DM. Main clinical	30 minutes 30 minutes 30 minutes	30 minutes 30 minutes 30 minutes	1 hour 1 hour 1 hour

manifestations that occur in CKD. **Second month**: Complications that occur in CKD. Measures to prevent it. **Third month**: Evaluation of the diabetic patients participating in the study is carried out,			

II. METHODOLOGICAL GUIDELINES

In order to achieve significant learning of the contents and objectives mentioned above, an educational programme is developed with several group sessions. Different active pedagogical techniques are used, such as expository techniques accompanied by discussion. The evaluation of the educational programme is carried out from the perspective of knowing whether the proposed objectives have been achieved and to determine whether the educational programme is successful. The evaluation is carried out during the whole process of intervention, before, during and at the end.

Prior to the implementation of the educational programme, a diagnostic questionnaire was used to obtain an individual diagnosis of learning needs.

During the application of the educational programme, the evaluation of the process is participatory as an active subject, by means of self-evaluation procedures in each session, and at the end of the educational activity, the evaluative questionnaire is applied to assess the level of information obtained.

The educational actions are based on five main thematic axes addressed in two stages, an intensive stage with 5 sessions and a reinforcement stage with 3 sessions. The activities will have a duration of one hour each and a fortnightly frequency. The place chosen is the 28 de Enero primary school, which is located within the radius of action of the family medical offices involved in the study, thus facilitating access and participation of the participating older adults.

Session 1: "Getting to know my illness".

Topic 1: Introduction to the educational programme: "Protecting my health".

General information on DM.

Objectives

Create a favourable state of mind and motivate the group to create a suitable atmosphere to raise interest in the topic to be discussed.

Define the methodology to be followed.

Establish general group norms and rules.

To know the general facts about diabetes mellitus.

The objectives are fulfilled in order to form the group, for which the members are introduced, creating a climate of interaction-participation through the techniques to be used.

Content:

Presentation of the educational activity to be developed.

DM. Concept. Symptoms. Complications. Control of the disease. Procedure:

Time: 1 hour.
Organisational form: Workshop.
Participatory technique: Presentation in pairs.
Media: Computer, blackboard, marker board and flipcharts.
Development of the activity:
The activity to be carried out is discussed with the diabetic patients, the aspects related to the research are discussed, taking into account objectives, stages, topics to be developed, duration.
Participants are introduced to each other and affective relationships are created between them.
The opening begins with the technique of presentation in pairs.
Afterwards, the participants are shown pictures and asked some questions about the topic. After this, the subject matter is explained.
Group reflection techniques and collective debate on what has been learned in the activity and its usefulness are carried out.
The closing of the activity is done by each participant stating whether "I help myself or not" for my future life.
Evaluation: the P.N.I. (Positive, Negative and Interesting) technique will be used.
Session 2: "How can I get sick? "
Topic 2: Risk factors that may cause CKD in patients with type 2 DM.
Objectives
To know what CKD is and its relationship with DM.
Explain the risk factors that may cause CKD in patients with type 2 DM.
Content
ERC. Concept. General overview of the disease.
Non-modifiable risk factors that may cause CKD in diabetic patients.
Modifiable risk factors that may cause CKD in diabetic patients.
Procedure:
Time: 1 hour.
Organisational form: Workshop.
Participatory technique: "Brainstorming".
Media: Computer, whiteboard, marker board and flip charts.
Development of the activity:
An exchange takes place for participants to discuss what happened in the previous meeting.
Then, orientation is given on the activity to be carried out.
In the first step, a pleasant conversation is held about the risk factors for CKD, and knowledge of the subject is explored.
Using the brainstorming technique, diabetic patients present their views on the cause of the onset of CKD, define the risks and highlight the importance of knowing them for general health.
Afterwards, the participants are divided into two groups, handed out flip charts and folders, which contain images of different types of situations so that the participants can classify them as risks or not.
At the end of this part, the risk factors for CKD in diabetic patients are classified into modifiable and non-modifiable risk factors.

A group technique is used in which the influence of this aspect on each of the participants is presented and the group concludes with an updated summary of the problem.

The activity ends with the dynamic "I'm going on a trip". It is about imagining that we are going on a trip and we say something of ours that we would like to take with us or something that we would like to give to our partner. All participants have to sit on a circle. Then the first participant starts by saying "I'm going on a trip and I'm taking a smile with me" and has to smile to the person on his or her right. Then that person has to say "I'm going on a trip and I'm taking a smile and a hug" and gives the person on his or her right a hug and a smile. Each person has to repeat what has been said and then add Evaluation:

The PNI (Positive, Negative, Interesting) is applied to find out the opinion of the group on the actions carried out.

Session 3: "What can I feel?

Topic 3: Main clinical manifestations occurring in CKD. Objective

Identify the main clinical manifestations that occur in CKD.

Content

CKD. Main clinical manifestations. Procedure:

Time: 1 hour.

Organisational form: Workshop.

Participatory technique: "Fears and hope".

Means: Computer, blackboard, marker board and flipcharts Development of the activity:

The "fears and hopes" technique is used to establish a conversational relationship between the professional and the older adults to discuss the main clinical manifestations that can occur in patients with CKD. Subsequently, any concerns they may have on the subject are collected on the blackboard and a debate is held to reinforce their level of information.

All participants are seated in a circle, from left to right, each one says a nice word or phrase to the other, then from right to left the one who gave affection receives it and then this is expressed out loud for all to hear.

Evaluation: the P.N.I. (Positive, Negative and Interesting) technique is used to obtain the criteria of each participant.

Session 4: "Recognising the danger".

Topic 4: Complications occurring in CKD.

Target

Explain the complications that can occur after the occurrence of CKD.

Content

CKD. Major complications.

Procedure

Time: 1 hour.

Organisational form: Workshop.

Participatory technique: "Agree - disagree".

Media: Computer, whiteboard, marker board and flipcharts Activity Development

Information on the subject is presented by the specialist.

The technique: "Agree - disagree" is used to show the diabetic patients participating

in the study the complications that can occur in the event of developing CKD. Examples of fictitious situations reflecting these conditions are used for reflection and discussion.
Group reflection techniques and collective debate on what has been learnt in the activity are carried out.
The activity is concluded with the affective technique "Stimulating phrases", which aims to stimulate self-confidence related to avoiding the complications that arise in CKD and to promote a satisfactory emotional state in the group. A strip of paper is made for each member of the group and a sentence is written on each one. They are placed in a small box and chosen at random. Each participant reads their sentences with emphasis.
Evaluation: the P.N.I. (Positive, Negative and Interesting) technique is used to obtain the criteria of each participant.
Session 5: "I am preparing myself to improve my health".
Topic 5: Measures to prevent CKD.
Target
To outline preventive measures for the occurrence of CKD. Content
CKD. Main measures to prevent their occurrence. Procedure
Time: 1 hour.
Organisational form: Workshop.
Participatory technique: "Rotate debate".
Media: Computer, whiteboard, marker board and flipcharts Activity Development
The author makes a commentary on what was covered in the previous session and the knowledge acquired up to this session and any doubts that may arise regarding the subject are discussed. To continue the activity, the "Rotate debate" technique is applied with the aim of examining a problem from multiple angles. Subsequently, all possible preventive measures in the occurrence of chronic kidney disease are explained in a clear and simple way, using the blackboard.
The activity is dismissed with the technique: "An orchestra without instruments". Explain to the group that they are "part of an orchestra" but that the orchestra has no instruments. The orchestra will not be able to say any words, but only use sounds that can be made with the human body like clapping, humming, whistling, etc. Following this, each participant must choose a sound and you will ask them to play a song that is familiar to the group.
Evaluation: The P.N.I. (Positive, Negative and Interesting) technique will be used.
Reinforcement stage
Theme: "What to learn^ about the ERC".
Duration: A monthly meeting for three months.
Objective:
To assess the level of information about CKD acquired by diabetic patients participating in the educational programme.
Content:
Month 1: General information on DM and CKD. Risk factors that can cause CKD in diabetic patients. Main clinical manifestations that occur in CKD.
Second month: Complications that occur in CKD.
Measures to prevent it.

Third month: Evaluation of the diabetic patients participating in the study is carried out.

Procedure for the first and second month.

Time: 1 hour.

Organisational form: Workshop.

Media: Slides, videos, computer, sheets, pens.

Development of the first and second month's activities:

Start with the orientation of the activity, then sitting in a circle, the participants explain their favourite activities and the reasons for their preferences.

The researcher conducts an exchange of ideas on each topic as appropriate, the participants contribute their criteria, ideas are clarified, practical activities on the current topics are carried out and conclusions are drawn.

Feedback is given at the end of the interventions and the actions to be taken by the participants at each meeting are organised.

Third month: Closing and final evaluation:

Objective.

To verify that the diabetic patients were able to adapt to the educational messages conveyed.

To evaluate the modifications in the level of knowledge at individual and group level after the application of the educational actions.

Content.

Reaffirmation of theoretical contents and acquired skills. Procedure.

Time: 1 hour

Organisational form: Integrative workshop

Media: Computer, whiteboard, marker board and flip charts.

Development of the activity

The activity begins with the "fortune biscuit" dynamic, followed by an exchange and discussion activity with the diabetic patients in which there is a conversation and dialogue related to the way in which the participants were able to deal with the topics taught. An integrative workshop is held to summarise the most significant aspects found during the application of the educational actions, seeking feedback on the positive and negative aspects.

Once the execution of the educational actions is finished, an evaluation questionnaire is applied to the older adults with the same questions that were asked in the initial questionnaire, which allows to verify what has been learned and finally to compare with the results obtained in the initial diagnosis.

Participants are encouraged to think of a word that describes what they learned during their participation in the educational actions. They are given a few minutes to do so. Each participant says that word without reflecting on it.

The patients with the highest participation during the development of the educational actions are recognised.

It concludes with a farewell tea.

DESCRIPTION OF THE PARTICIPATING TECHNIQUES

Technique: Presentation in pairs.

Target

S Making the presentations of the teacher and participants of the programme.

Development

The facilitator gives the indication that we are going to introduce ourselves in pairs and that they should exchange certain information that is of interest to everyone, e.g. name, interest in the course, expectations, information about their job, where they come from and some personal information. Each person finds a partner he/she does not know and they talk for five minutes. Then, in assembly, each participant introduces his/her partner. The duration of this dynamic will depend on the number of participants, usually a maximum of three minutes per pair is given to each participant. the presentation in plenary

Technique: "Brainstorming

Objective:

Get the whole group to contribute ideas or thoughts on the information they have on the topic.

Development

The facilitator starts the activity by asking the group an open question related to the topic developed during the session. Subsequently, the participants are asked to contribute their ideas on the question posed. Once the production of ideas has been exhausted, the ideas are ordered and organised in order to create a system of interrelationships with which to explain the problem or theme that is the focus of the study.

Dynamics "I'm going on a trip".

It is about imagining that we are going on a trip and saying something of ours that we would like to take with us or something that we would like to give to our partner.

Target

To favour the affirmation and cohesion of the group.

Development

All participants should sit in a circle. Then you say: "I'm going on a trip and I'm taking a smile with me" and you should smile at the person on your right. Then that person has to say "I'm going on a trip and I'm taking a smile and a hug" and gives the person on his or her right a hug and a smile. Each person has to repeat what has been said and then add a new action to the list. Continue in this way^ until everyone has participated.

Technique: "Fears and Hopes".

Objective:

Raise the group's awareness of their motivations, desires and hopes, anxieties and fears.

Development

This consists of each of the patients stating their fears and hopes about the topic discussed, followed by a summary of what they consider to be the main factors that were discussed.

Technique "Giving and receiving affection.

Objective:

Experiencing the problems related to giving and receiving affection.

It is a technique that allows you to recognise actions that harm or benefit others and how it feels to help someone. It allows you to be able to ask for, receive and offer help, and to explain the emotions that arise when supporting and being supported.

An activity that promotes integration between team members and builds trust between them.

Development

All participants seated in a circle, from left to right, each said a nice word or phrase to each other, then from right to left the one who gave appreciation received it and then this was expressed aloud for all to hear.

Technique: "Agree - disagree".

Objective:

Define individual and team positions in relation to a series of statements determined by the coordinator.

Development

The coordinator presents the group with a series of statements and asks them to silently and individually indicate whether they agree or disagree with each of them, divides the group into small teams and gives them the following instructions: "The job of each team is to decide, by consensus, whether they agree or disagree with each of these statements. They should not decide by majority vote, but through discussion and substantiation of opinions.

Technique: Stimulating phrases

Objective:

Stimulate self-confidence.

Development

Make a strip of paper for each member of the group and write a sentence on each one. They are placed in a small box and chosen at random. Each participant reads their sentences with emphasis.

Dynamics Rotating Debates

Objectives

Explore the different arguments that can be constructed from different perspectives.

Encourage debate as a good social practice.

Rethinking and reflecting on ideas

Development

The Rotating Debates dynamic is an activity that uses a variety of scenarios to encourage critical thinking. More importantly, the ability to examine a problem from multiple angles.

The exercise co-ordinator should form two teams to discuss and present them with an issue that is problematic. The issue can be broad and wide-ranging, such as climate change; or narrow and interpersonal, such as a conflict over the use of resources in an office.

Each team should be assigned a side of the conflict, which they will then discuss for 2-3 minutes, with the facilitator ordering the discussion. Once each side has made its point, switch sides and have each team argue the counterpoint.

Technique : "An orchestra without instruments.

Target

Promote disinhibition and generate a relaxed group atmosphere.

Contributing to group interaction

Development

You should explain to the group that they are "part of an orchestra", however, the orchestra has no instruments. The orchestra will not be able to say any words, but will only use sounds that can be made with the human body such as clapping, humming, whistling, etc. Following this, each participant must choose a sound and will be asked to play a song that is familiar to the group.

Technique: "PNI" (positive, negative, interesting)

Allow participants to give their opinions about the positive, negative and interesting aspects of the activities carried out. It can be done orally, but it is advisable for participants to write down their opinions on sheets of paper and then analyse them as a group and write a report.

Fortune Cookie Dynamics

Objectives

Facilitate the farewell between the members of a common space.

Promote the expression of mutual desires.

Leaving a space by leaving encouraging words

Development

Fortune biscuits are small biscuits that contain a paper with a message inside. This message is considered to be the fortune or luck of the person who breaks the biscuit and reads it.

This activity aims to imitate the fortune or luck message of the biscuits. Participants should be told what fortune biscuits are all about.

Each participant is given a few minutes to write a brief wish and/or omen. This should be a message addressed to the whole group.

For example you can write "I wish that what we have learnt can be put into practice successfully". The coordinator will collect all the messages and mix them in a bag.

At random, each member takes a piece of paper from the bag and reads the message out loud as if it were an affirmation. As they read it they personalise it, e.g. "what I have learnt I will be able to put into practice successfully".

BIBLIOGRAPHICAL REFERENCES

1. Tejada-Tayabas LM, Pastor-Durango MP, Gutierrez-Enriquez SO. Effectiveness of an educational program in the control of patients with diabetes. Invest Educ Enferm [Internet] 2006 [cited 2024 my 26]; 24 (2): 48-53. Available from: https://www.redalyc.org/pdf/1052/105215402004.pdf

2. Dunlay SM, Givertz MM, Aguilar D, Allen LA, Chan M, Desai AS, et al. Type 2 diabetes mellitus and heart failure: a Scientifics tatement fromthe American HeartAssociation andthe Heart Failure Society of America: thisstatementdoesnotrepresentupdateofthe 2017 ACC/AHA/HFSA heartfailureguidelineupdate. "Circulation [Internet] 2019 [cited 2024 my 26]; 140 (7) e294-e324. Available from: https://doi: 10.1161/CIR.0000000000000691. Epub 2019 Jun 6. Erratum in: Circulation. 2019 Sept 17; 140(12):e692. PMID: 31167558.

3. Aldrete-Velasco J, Chiquete E, Rodriguez-Garrta J, Rincon PR, Correa RR, Garrta PR, et al. Mortality from chronic kidney disease and its relationship with diabetes in Mexico. Med Interna Mex [Internet] 2018 Jul-Aug [cited 2024 my 26]; 34(4): 536-550. Available from: https://doi.org/10.24245/mim.v34i4.1877

4. Chipi-Cabrera JA, Fernandini-Escalona E. Chronic kidney disease presumptive in older adults. Rev Colomb Nefrol [Internet] 2019 Jul-Dec

[cited2024my26]; 6(2): 138-151. Available from: Rev Colomb Nefrol [Internet] 2019 Jul-Dec [cited2024my26]; 6(2): 138-151 . in: https://doi.org/10.22265/acnef.6.2.352

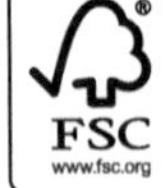

MIX
Papier aus verantwortungsvollen Quellen
Paper from responsible sources
FSC® C105338

Printed by Books on Demand GmbH, Norderstedt / Germany